"This engaging book is spot on. I am most impressed. The research Dr Falck has done, in the literature and her own research, is phenomenal. She gives many telling examples, and illustrates her points most convincingly. It has given me sheer joy to read this and witness this particular cheetah running free. It will be ages before this book ceases to surpass all others in this important field: it deserves to do extremely well."

– **Patrick Casement, British Psychoanalytical Society, UK**

"Dr Falck's book is of singular importance for adults with exceptional intelligence and clinicians who work with them therapeutically. She places her data, observations, suggestions, and conclusions in the context of an extensive literature review, making her book comprehensive and up to date. It is an authentic, stimulating, and impressive resource that contributes a deeper understanding of the interpersonal psychology of exceptionally intelligent individuals. Her research interviews with very high-IQ adults should in themselves help similar others 'normalise' the social dynamics they experience that unfortunately can so often be confusing and disappointing or worse. This book should inspire further pursuit of more adaptive solutions and help reverse the trend of denying, disavowing, or deconstructing the remarkable asset that extreme intelligence can be. This is a compellingly written work that makes a major contribution to this field."

– **Dr Jerald Grobman, Distinguished Fellow of the American Psychiatric Association, USA**

EXTREME INTELLIGENCE

Extreme intelligence is strongly correlated with the highest of human achievement, but also, paradoxically, with higher relationship conflict, career difficulty, mental illness, and high-IQ crime. Increased intelligence does not necessarily increase success; it should be considered as a minority special need that requires nurturing.

This book explores the social development and predicaments of those who possess extreme intelligence, and the consequent personal and professional implications for them. It uniquely integrates insights and knowledge from the research fields of intelligence, giftedness, genius, and expertise with those from depth psychology, emphasising the importance of finding ways to talk effectively about extreme intelligence, and how it can better be supported and embraced. The author supports her arguments throughout, reviewing the academic literature alongside representations of genius in history, fiction, and the media, and draws on her own first-hand research interviews and consulting work with multinational high-IQ adults.

This book is essential reading for anyone supporting or working with the highly gifted, as well as those researching or interested by the field of intelligence.

Dr Sonja Falck is a Senior Lecturer at the School of Psychology, University of East London, UK. She is also a UKCP and BACP accredited psychotherapist and supervisor. She consults in person and online internationally, specialising in high-ability adults' relationship issues. She has presented at SENG (Supporting the Emotional Needs of the Gifted), USA, and the British branch of the international high IQ society Mensa.

EXTREME INTELLIGENCE

Development, Predicaments, Implications

Sonja Falck

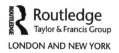

LONDON AND NEW YORK

First published 2020
by Routledge
2 Park Square, Milton Park, Abingdon, Oxon OX14 4RN

and by Routledge
52 Vanderbilt Avenue, New York, NY 10017

Routledge is an imprint of the Taylor & Francis Group, an informa business

© 2020 Sonja Falck

The right of Sonja Falck to be identified as author of this work has been asserted by them in accordance with sections 77 and 78 of the Copyright, Designs and Patents Act 1988.

All rights reserved. No part of this book may be reprinted or reproduced or utilised in any form or by any electronic, mechanical, or other means, now known or hereafter invented, including photocopying and recording, or in any information storage or retrieval system, without permission in writing from the publishers.

Trademark notice: Product or corporate names may be trademarks or registered trademarks, and are used only for identification and explanation without intent to infringe.

British Library Cataloguing-in-Publication Data
A catalogue record for this book is available from the British Library

Library of Congress Cataloging-in-Publication Data
A catalog record has been requested for this book

ISBN: 978-1-138-61334-8 (hbk)
ISBN: 978-1-138-61335-5 (pbk)
ISBN: 978-0-429-46453-9 (ebk)

Typeset in Bembo
by Swales & Willis, Exeter, Devon, UK

Printed and bound by CPI Group (UK) Ltd, Croydon, CR0 4YY

This book is dedicated, in the order in which I got to know them, to:

Dan (in memoriam) & Queda
Colin
Damon
Lawrence
Richard

CONTENTS

Extended table of contents — xi
List of illustrations — xvi
Acknowledgements — xvii
Preface: mother says no — xix

Introduction: how do we think and speak about extreme intelligence? — 1

PART I
Development — 11

1 Measures and methods: the identifying and quantifying of intelligence — 13

2 The roots of difference: how is it that some people stand out so much from others? — 31

3 Core biopsychosocial issues: needing to be noticed, dreading rejection — 51

PART II
Predicaments — 71

4 Recognition and reactions: what happens when someone stands out so much? — 73

5 Naive Child, Arrogant Emperor: are the intellectually adept, socially inept?   95

6 Madness, misunderstanding, and misdiagnosis: is extreme intelligence a benefit or a liability?   115

PART III
Implications   139

7 Entrapment: the unintentional perpetuation of interpersonal trouble   141

8 Hiding Self, Reaching Out: the "High-IQ Relational Styles" framework   154

9 Helping high ability thrive: channelling abilities whilst managing threat   173

Conclusion: implications for the world around us   195

Appendix: explaining the research process that underpins the book   200

Index   *209*

EXTENDED TABLE OF CONTENTS

Preface: mother says no   xix

Introduction: how do we think and speak about extreme intelligence?   1

    An extreme on the Bell Curve 1
    The language of intelligence and related concepts 3
    Use of research 5
    The book's scope, focus, and originality 7
    Structure of the book 8
    The Reflective Prompts at the start of each chapter 8

PART I
Development   11

1 Measures and methods: the identifying and quantifying of intelligence   13

    The difficulty of talking about intelligence 14
    Understanding the controversy 15
    The academic literature's definitions and theories of intelligence 17
        Spearman's g 19
        The Cattell–Horn theory of fluid and crystallised intelligences 19
        Gardner's multiple intelligences 19
        Sternberg's theory of successful intelligence 20
    Is there ever any good reason to try to measure intelligence? 20

Can intelligence actually be measured? 21
Quantifying genius 24
Identifying extreme intelligence and intelligence generally in everyday life 25

2 The roots of difference: how is it that some people stand out so much from others? 31

The nature versus nurture debate 32
    Practise and expertise 33
    Individual difference 33
    Social and interpersonal implications 34
    Factors in combination 35
The trajectory of intelligence research: where it has been and where it might go 37
    What produces intelligence? 39
    Who has it? 41
    How stable or changeable is intelligence? 42
    Attempts to increase intelligence: genetic, environmental, augmentative? 43
An analogy encapsulating the main issues 45

3 Core biopsychosocial issues: needing to be noticed, dreading rejection 51

The "High-IQ Context" model 51
Goals: survival, belonging, competition, collaboration 52
Recognition: the interpersonal mirror that establishes self-esteem 55
Person: the extremely high-IQ individual 56
    Biological basis 56
    Experiential and behavioural characteristics 57
    Minority status 57
    Goals revisited 58
Environment: country, culture, family, school, workplace 60
Person–environment reciprocal recognition and interaction 60
Moving between environments: transferring habits and expectations 63
Three kinds of change 65

PART II
Predicaments 71

4 Recognition and reactions: what happens when someone stands out so much? 73

Comparing and competing 74

Being recognised by others 75
Recognising something about yourself: effort and speed 78
Being set apart versus belonging 81
Problems surrounding differentials in effort 85
From the classroom to the courtroom 88
The dynamics of envy: a compassion barrier 90

5 Naive Child, Arrogant Emperor: are the intellectually adept, socially inept?   95

The stereotype of the extremely intelligent person as socially inept 96
The academic literature: asserting versus denying interpersonal difficulties 97
Causes: how difficulty arises 100
Nature of the difficulty: two main kinds 101
    The "Naive Child" profile 104
    The "Arrogant Emperor" profile 105
    Differences and connections between the two profiles 106
Consequences of interpersonal difficulties 107
Impact on individuals' prospects of actualising their potential 108
Reasons for the stereotype 109

6 Madness, misunderstanding, and misdiagnosis: is extreme intelligence a benefit or a liability?   115

Is having the highest possible intelligence best? 116
Genius, madness, creativity 118
Misdiagnosis 121
Naive Child and autism 122
Arrogant Emperor and narcissism 127
Aetiological similarities 129
Benefit, liability, and relational influences 132

PART III
Implications   139

7 Entrapment: the unintentional perpetuation of interpersonal trouble   141

The past in the present 142
Challenging transference 145
Valency 148
Repetition compulsion 149
Change, and resistance to change 151

8 Hiding Self, Reaching Out: the "High-IQ Relational Styles" framework — 154

Introducing and explaining the framework 155
Hiding Self 156
    Top left quadrant: Inhibited 156
    Bottom left quadrant: Despairing 158
Reaching Out 159
    Bottom right quadrant: Provoking 159
    Top right quadrant: Thriving 161
Moving between quadrants 162
Linking High-IQ Relational Styles with other giftedness life-strategies/trajectories 163
Congruences with other psychological thinking 165
    Recognition revisited 166
    Further considerations regarding Attachment Theory and Object Relations 167

9 Helping high ability thrive: channelling abilities whilst managing threat — 173

Parenting and schooling 174
    Identification 174
    Resources 175
    Strategies: safeguarding against naivety and arrogance 176
In the workplace: facilitating collaboration and competition 178
Revisiting High-IQ Relational Styles: change towards "Thriving" 181
    Changing the nature of the environment 183
    Change in the interface between self and environment 184
    Professional consultancy resources: therapy, coaching 187
    Optimising personal performance 189
What is success? 190

Conclusion: implications for the world around us — 195

Appendix: explaining the research process that underpins the book — 200

Summary of Constructivist Grounded Theory (CGT) procedures 200
Data collection 201
Quality control 201
Analysing the data 201
Memo writing 202
Constructing theory 203

A Psychosocial interpretation of the data 205
Theoretical sampling 205
Limitations 206
Wider applications 206

Index 209

ILLUSTRATIONS

Figures

0.1	The Bell Curve of human intelligence	2
0.2	Potential and performance	4
1.1	History of influences in the development of intelligence theory and testing	18
2.1	Intelligence Research schema	37
3.1	High-IQ Context model	52
3.2	Three kinds of change	66
6.1	Child and Emperor: naivety and arrogance in interpersonal relating	131
8.1	High-IQ Relational Styles framework	155
9.1	Change towards "Thriving"	182
A.1	High-IQ Context model with research data focused codes and theoretical categories	204

Tables

3.1	Manifestations of very high IQ	58
5.1	Distinguishing Naive Child versus Arrogant Emperor characteristics of interpersonal relating	106
8.1	High-IQ Relational Styles and other authors' giftedness life-strategies/trajectories	164
A.1	Research data focused codes	202
A.2	Research data focused codes and theoretical categories	204

ACKNOWLEDGEMENTS

I am grateful to my research interviewees, colleagues, and clients who have given their permission for me to use material from our conversations, and to the Metanoia Institute and British Mensa for their involvement in the foundational stages of this project. I thank my University of East London colleagues for their much appreciated support, particularly Dr Lucia Berdondini for her incredible kindness; Dr Yannis Fronimos; Max Eames for his critique of the final draft of the manuscript; and Dr Elley Wakui who gave input on statistics. My thanks to Damon Falck for assistance with graphics and for our enjoyable conversations that helped me refine my Intelligence Research schema and computer analogy. Thanks to Zea Eagle for her original artwork and the process of collaboration involved. I am grateful to Patrick Casement and Dr Jerald Grobman for their endorsements. For other forms of support, I thank Esther Graumann, Chris Edwards and Sandra Goldsack and my reliably attentive editors at Routledge, Ceri McLardy and Sophie Crowe. My special thanks to Tony Noguera and Christa Gonschorrek who rescued the book during exceptionally challenging times by so generously initiating and providing for me an unforgettable writing retreat. Thank you to Dr Colin Falck and Lawrence Falck for their unfailing daily close involvement and many sacrifices that enabled me to keep writing, and to Richard Harding for his faithful patience and support.

I am grateful for the following permissions:

- In Chapter 2 (p. 31), the words from Caroline Lawrence's novel *The Roman Mysteries: The Enemies of Jupiter*, have been reproduced by permission of Orion Children's Books, an imprint of Hachette Children's Group, Carmelite House, 50 Victoria Embankment, London, EC4Y 0DZ.

- In Chapter 5 (p. 96), the words from *The Ogre of Oglefort*, Eva Ibbotson and Alex T. Smith 2010, have been reproduced by permission of Macmillan Children's Books.
- This is the agreed copyright line for the words in Chapter 5 (p. 96) used from *Harry Potter and the Philosopher's Stone*: Copyright © J. K. Rowling 1997.

PREFACE: MOTHER SAYS NO

When I was seven, growing up in South Africa, my schoolteacher called my mother in. It was explained that they wanted to send me to "a university programme for gifted children". My mother said no. "Sonja can't have a conversation with figures," she asserted (and repeated many times over the years whenever she retold the story), "or marry a book." She recommended that when I finished my work way ahead of the rest of the class, the teacher should occupy me by using me to help the others. My mother was proud of her decision, always depicting it as having saved me from becoming a social outcast.

Decades and continents away from this moment, my firstborn child was at his school in London identified as gifted. Suddenly I was the mother with responsibility for making decisions about this that I knew would impact his whole future. I realised that in all the intervening time I had never even found out what this term "gifted" actually meant. What I also realised, was that my mother's words to my teacher revealed at least three assumptions: 1. That this thing called giftedness was associated with social difficulty; 2. That relationships were of primary importance (which included seeing marriage as the priority future to secure for a daughter); 3. That it was best to try to keep an apparently gifted child (and perhaps particularly if female?) looking as normal as possible, without special provision being made to engage with her abilities: being "normal" rather than "gifted" was best. I realised that these attitudes – or, one could say, these prejudices or fears – had left me with an implicit message that I could only not become a pariah by not fully developing my own capabilities. Where did this assumption come from, I began to wonder, of an association between giftedness and social difficulty? By this point I was a well-established psychotherapist – yes, I'd been helping others all my life (and, moreover, through a medium that emphasises the importance of relationship) – but I had some restlessness around feeling I was not using my full potential. I commenced a doctorate through which I began to research these questions.

What I found was that one objectively measurable aspect of those who come to be termed gifted is that they can usually achieve an extremely high score on a standardised IQ test (this is explained in the Introduction and critically discussed in Chapter 1). I also found that how best to deal with the schooling of a child of this kind is internationally a challenging and controversial issue that fills several journals, conferences, and books. And I found that whether such children grow up to use their "full potential" was also a well-documented issue. Whilst there is representation in the literature of issues such as genetic heritability and the effects of gender and culture on how manifestations of high intelligence are responded to, what is less represented is the inheritance of related attitudes and implicit messages that are repeated from one generation to the next. For example, what implicit messages had my mother picked up about this, that informed how she reacted when she was called in by my teacher? The way she dealt with her meeting with my teacher transmitted messages that were unconsciously absorbed by me, and without me stopping to examine this more carefully – as I did only many years later – such messages would have determined how I would handle this with my own children. Which they in turn would pass on. And so on and on this could go (and usually does). Through my research I encountered many, many moving stories of families who had had to make decisions in the face of an identification of giftedness, with long-term impact.

Most intriguing of all for me, however, was that through my research I found that there was indeed in relation to extreme intelligence a ubiquitous presence of a concern about social difficulty. I also observed that this was an issue that was not in any one resource comprehensively explored, and certainly not at the depth a psychotherapist would find satisfactory. The aim of this book, therefore, is to provide such a resource.

The book engages with the topic of extreme intelligence (and related concepts such as giftedness, expertise, and genius, which will be explained) from the angle of emphasising how the perennial fascination with and typical reactions to this topic shape the social development of individuals with very high IQ and cause various predicaments. In the course of this it also addresses the contemporary concern with how to think about, produce, and handle manifestations of excellence. I review the relevant academic literature; present excerpts from my research interviews with very high-IQ individuals; draw on my consulting work (psychotherapy and coaching) with high-IQ clients as well as my experience as a university lecturer and a parent; and refer to representations of extreme intelligence in history, novels, and the media. This book is relevant for you if you are in any way interested in or affected by this topic. I hope you will enjoy reading it and find in it something worthwhile to discover.

INTRODUCTION

How do we think and speak about extreme intelligence?

The titles of this book's introduction and conclusion explicitly state its overarching theme: how do we think about, speak about, and relate to extreme intelligence; and what are the implications of this for affected individuals and the world around us? Here "extreme" refers to the upper extreme of the Bell Curve of human intelligence. I will begin with a foundational explanation of the statistical practices used in what has been the predominant method of trying to quantify human intelligence. This will show how rare what I am calling extreme intelligence is and how significantly it stands out within a general population.

An extreme on the Bell Curve

The predominant way of representing different levels of human intelligence is by referring to numerical values derived from scores obtained on IQ tests (this will be critically discussed in Chapter 1). How this works is that large numbers of people are administered a standardised IQ test, meaning all candidates answer the same questions under the same conditions and all tests are scored in the same way. The tests are designed to contain equal numbers of easy, average, and difficult questions.

When all these test scores are plotted on a graph, what is found is that the scores are distributed symmetrically around a mid-point, that mid-point being the score that is most frequently obtained (statistically termed the mode). A line drawn tracing along the top of the graph forms the shape of an inverted bell, hence such a distribution of data, which is called a Gaussian curve, is also called a Bell Curve. In such a distribution, 68% of the scores fall within one standard deviation of the mode ("standard deviation" refers to how much variation there is within a distribution of data). Such a distribution of data is also called a normal distribution. Many sets of data taken from general human populations – such as

2 Introduction

measurements of height and blood pressure – follow this pattern. It allows one to see what the probability is of any particular score in the general population.

With IQ test scores the mode is set at 100, with the value of standard deviation set at 15. The most common IQ score is therefore 100, and the fact that the majority of IQ scores fall within one standard deviation of the mode means that the majority of IQ scores fall between 85 and 115. This is the Bell Curve of human intelligence (see Figure 0.1).

IQ is a relative rather than an absolute measure: it measures how people score in relation to each other. Looking at the left side of the Bell Curve, we can see that a minority of fewer than 3% of people score lower than 70 on an IQ test. Such a score would define a person as having an intellectual disability (British Psychological Society 2001; American Psychiatric Association 2013). Identified intellectual disability – usually referred to as learning disability in the UK – makes a person eligible for various kinds of assistance. In the UK this means eligibility for state-funded social skills training, supported housing, supported employment, and criminal justice liaison and diversion (meaning that how crime is judged and dealt with is handled differently when very low IQ is involved) (Parkin et al. 2018).

Moving to the right side of the Bell Curve, we see that there is similarly a small minority of fewer than 3% of people who achieve an IQ score of 130 or higher. It is this range of 130 and higher (indicated in bold on Figure 0.1) that I am referring to with the term "extreme intelligence". It is also this range that in academic research is identified with the term "gifted" (with some sources starting the range at slightly different points). In the USA it is a score of 130 or higher on the commonly used Stanford-Binet or Weschler intelligence tests that would gain a child admission to gifted educational programmes (Grobman 2017). A person with a score of 130 is two standard deviations away from the mode. Such a score is said to be on the 98th percentile, meaning that it is higher than what 98% of other test takers have scored. As scores get higher they

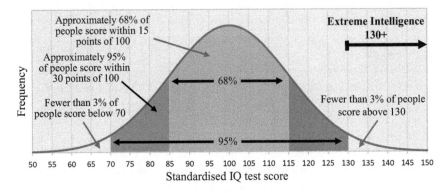

FIGURE 0.1 The Bell Curve of human intelligence.

become even more rare. Individuals with such scores are having to navigate a world which is generally as ill-adapted for their needs as it is for those who are intellectually disabled, although this is not typically recognised and there is certainly no state-funded assistance to support the adjustment of extremely high-IQ individuals. The psychosocial implications of this are what this book is concerned with.

Intelligence is a term that has overlaps with terms such as giftedness, high ability, talent, genius, and expertise, but – whereas these terms are hard to define precisely – the term extreme intelligence gives an objectively quantifiable focus of IQ that is measured on standardised tests to be at the 98th percentile or higher – in other words IQs in the top 2% of the population or higher. The word "extreme" also elicits connotations of "too much", "out of control", the idea that extremes are dangerous, that keeping within "safe limits" is what is mostly desired and advised. In terms of the Bell Curve, those whose IQ scores fall within the 68% majority referred to above are what constitute the norm, or the average. Whilst fitting within this "safe zone" – and within the extended 95% majority shown on Figure 0.1 – has its attractions, extremes are always alluring. We are intrigued by cases of extremes, as cautionary tales of the kinds of tragedies to beware of, or as fantasies of the kinds of success that can magnificently impress.

The language of intelligence and related concepts

In general conversation people usually have a colloquially shared grasp of what "intelligence" means, and of what it is in their experience of others that they would describe as intelligence. Two important components of this are questions of potential and of performance. Performance is what we can observe in a person – for example the way that the person speaks, writes, solves a problem, kicks a football, or plays a musical instrument. How proficiently, or not, these things are carried out, is often described in terms of how intelligent the performer is perceived as being. Intelligence is therefore a kind of potential that we impute to people, as an abstract phenomenon that underlies, and powers, their performance, making it possible for them to, for example, express themselves verbally or complete a mathematical calculation in the way that they do. We think of potential as being available to a person in greater or smaller quantities, but we cannot observe this directly – it is always an abstraction that we are inferring from their observable performance.

In Figure 0.2 I have arranged various intelligence-related terms according to whether I see them as relating primarily to the concept of potential (Circle 1), or to observable performance (Circle 2), or to both (the overlap between the two circles). A term such as "high ability", therefore, is in the overlap because it could denote either outstanding potential or outstanding performance, or a combination of the two. If you were arranging these terms, where would you place each one?

4 Introduction

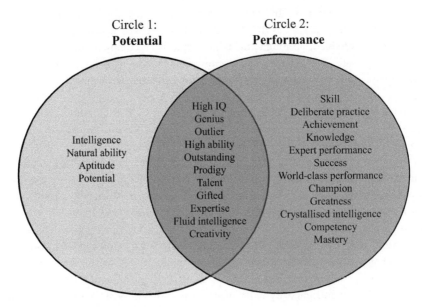

FIGURE 0.2 Potential and performance

Some of these terms come from specific theories and debates that will be encountered in subsequent chapters. There are whole books that focus on one or another of these terms, for example Syed (2010) focuses on what he calls "champions", Coyle (2010) on "talent", and Gladwell (2008) on "outliers". Different authors can be found to distinguish these terms differently, and could therefore differ from each other in how they would arrange the words in Figure 0.2. Some authors use the terms interchangeably. None that I have found give as comprehensive a definition of what they mean as Gagné (2013:193) does, who defines giftedness as "the possession and use of untrained and spontaneously expressed outstanding natural abilities or aptitudes (called gifts)", and talent as "the outstanding mastery of systematically developed competencies (knowledge and skills)". He defines "outstanding" as that which is within the top 10% of age peers, which is clearly a much broader range than the top 2% mentioned above. He goes into some detail about the "development process" that is involved in converting raw gifts into well-honed talents (Gagné 2013:193). So according to this, Gagné would put "gifted" in Figure 0.2's Circle 1 and "talented" in Circle 2, whilst I have placed both these terms in the overlap between the two circles. Some of these discrepancies are semantic, such as whether a term is being used as an adjective or a noun. Some terms have been hotly debated: the journal *Intelligence* even devoted a full volume (2014) to "expertise", with the gist of the debate being whether the term fits exclusively within Figure 0.2's Circle 2 or in the overlap between Circles 1 and 2. I have placed it in the overlap. I am not trying to provide a final definitive interpretation of these terms, but what I am trying to do is give an idea of the complexity involved, a complexity that should be kept in mind during your reading of this book.

Out of all these different terms, in order to access the largest stores of academic literature and research on extreme intelligence, apart from searching "intelligence" – and, more recently, "expertise", which has been developing a more substantial presence – the other most effective search term is "gifted". Although usages of the term gifted have been found dating back to 1825 (by Kearney 2009, cited in Silverman 2013), its origin is usually attributed to Sir Francis Galton, who first used it in 1869 in relation to children and adults who demonstrated exceptional ability in some area. The term has been in common use to refer to individuals of high potential certainly since the publication in 1926 of a book by Leta Hollingworth that included in its title the words "Gifted Children". I dislike the term "gifted" because – rather than it being a scientifically accurate and neutral term – it is judgement-laden and evokes unhelpful connotations of privilege. I will, however, unavoidably use the term throughout the book because there is so much literature and research on giftedness that is relevant to extreme intelligence given that, as mentioned, both terms relate to individuals whose IQ scores fall within the Bell Curve's far right tail. Giftedness, however, is not just about IQ score: individuals might not perform well on an IQ test but still match other descriptors of giftedness. This – termed twice exceptionality, or dual or multiple exceptionality – is introduced in Chapter 1.

Intelligence underpins so much of what is going on in the world around us. How we view it informs what we tell our children about what – and why – they and others can expect to achieve; how we design our educational systems; and how we run organisations. Yet it is something we do not readily or comfortably talk about. Reasons for this are presented in Chapter 1. Where the topic of intelligence is broached, people can be very opinionated about it, with specialists in the field having strong ideas of what is right or wrong or which aspects or issues are most important to focus on. I have even had peer reviewers declare which researchers and theorists within the field are the "correct" ones to refer to. The topic's emotiveness and controversy will be recognised and referred to as a presence to be taken into account throughout the book. In studying this topic, it becomes evident that different individuals, and groups, can be personally or politically invested in viewing things in one way or another. It is therefore worth asking ourselves, how do we *want* to think or speak about intelligence, and why?

Use of research

I uphold the ideal of keeping our thinking informed by rigorous research. However, I recognise that, rather than research being a resource that can provide reliable conclusions, it is often contradictory and comes with many problematic issues – particularly in an area as controversial and emotive as intelligence is – and that significant findings, especially if unpopular to commissioners of or consumers of research, can be slow to infiltrate a culture. For example, Haier (2017) documents how an enthusiasm for a belief that simply listening to Mozart could increase IQ – the "Mozart Effect" – persisted for 17 years in spite of research that disproved this, because of how much people wanted to believe that a benefit like this could be so easily accessible.

Some of the current challenges to approaching extreme intelligence scientifically are legacies of the field's ignominious history, as explained in Chapter 1. Other challenges relate to questions of what methodologies are used in data collection, interpretation, and dissemination. For example, a clear distortion in several studies on very high IQ is that the research participants were recruited from groups of already proven high achievers (such as the American Presidential Scholars programme). In such cases, findings that are presented as relating to individuals who have very high IQ are actually only true of individuals who have very high IQ *in addition to* having had access (geographically, socioeconomically, and educationally) to such programmes and *in addition to* having performed well enough by the programmes' criteria to have secured their places on such programmes. The complexity of matters to do with research is acknowledged throughout the book: examples are given of directly contradictory research findings and attention is drawn to specific issues on which research evidence has been unequivocal.

Almost all research in the field of intelligence is quantitative. This involves abstracting data from the individuals it is collected from, turning it into numbers and statistical products, and attempting to establish objective trends within or between groups of as many participants as possible. An alternative approach is qualitative research. This contributes a very different kind of data by paying close attention to individuals' own subjective experiences. It presents accounts of these and analyses and interprets them, finding themes and exploring meanings within and across such data. An example of the different contributions these different kinds of research can have, is that quantitative research has shown that very high-IQ people are less likely to have children (Meisenberg 2010). But why might this be? Qualitative research can start to fill in possible reasons. Favier-Townsend's (2014) interviews with a sample of British Mensa members revealed that most of them had chosen not to have children and had chosen this because their own childhood experiences of not having their intellectual needs understood or catered for were so miserable that they did not want to watch a child of their own going through that. They also wanted to avoid, through the process of raising a child, being faced with having to remember their own negative childhood experiences.

In this book I will be presenting original qualitative research I undertook, which included personal interviews with adults with very high IQ. The opportunity that the research interview afforded the participants to discuss confidentially and candidly the topic of extreme intelligence and how they were affected by it was repeatedly communicated to me as having been valued, with the words that were most often used to describe the interview experience being that it was found "interesting", "therapeutic", "thought-provoking", and "enjoyable". To protect the interviewees' anonymity they are referred to throughout by pseudonyms, and any other potentially identifying details have been omitted or obscured. Direct quotations from interviews are used, but for ease of reading the page numbers from the interview transcripts – which are available – are only included when showing how far apart from each other particular statements were made within the same interview. An Appendix is provided that elaborates my research process in further detail. Where I use material deriving from my consulting work (psychotherapy and coaching) with high-IQ clients, I have in the same way ensured anonymity. I obtained consent from interviewees and clients for using material from our conversations in anonymised form.

The book's scope, focus, and originality

I have found that there are four fields of research and scholarship relatively distinct from each other that relate to what are named respectively as intelligence, giftedness, expertise, and genius. This book uniquely draws on knowledge and insights from all of these fields. Additionally, this is integrated with knowledge and insights from the field of depth psychology, emphasising a relational perspective, in a way that I have not seen done before and that can hopefully be illuminating for readers involved in any of these fields or personally affected by the issues. It aims to be accessible to readers from diverse backgrounds and to stimulate personal reflection and interesting social and/or professional conversation. The book begins by introducing the main issues in the field of intelligence as these provide an important foundation and context for examining the related social dynamics. However, rather than simply documenting historical details in the study of intelligence, emphasis will be on their psychosocial implications.

The literature and research on giftedness overwhelmingly relates to children rather than adults and is predominantly focused on questions of how to deal with giftedness in school education. My focus is on the psychosocial aspects of extreme intelligence as encountered in adulthood, although this is affected by developmental experiences through childhood. Whilst education, twice exceptionality, culture, race, gender, and socioeconomics will all be mentioned as issues that can promote or hinder highly intelligent individuals, the overriding focus will be on the interpersonal interaction aspect. The way a parent, sibling, teacher, peer, employer, or practitioner reacts to an individual's manifestation of characteristics associated with high intelligence, and how the individual in turn responds, is what creates the interpersonal building blocks that underlie the way that various systems around us function (families, and educational and occupational organisations). It is with these underlying details and the patterns they establish that my main fascination lies. Arguably it is also with these details that any beneficial change in established patterns has to begin.

Structure of the book

The book is organised into three parts – Development, Predicaments, and Implications – with three chapters in each. Part I – Development – looks at the development of extreme intelligence in three main ways, one per chapter: firstly (Chapter 1), as a concept and psychological construct that has developed a related history and field of enquiry; secondly (Chapter 2), as a phenomenon that develops within certain individuals in a way that makes them stand out from others; and thirdly (Chapter 3), as something extraordinary that co-exists with ordinary general human lifespan development.

Part II – Predicaments – delves with increasing layers of complexity into explaining and exploring the various social predicaments that very high-IQ individuals often encounter and grapple with: Chapter 4 looks at the typical intrapersonal and interpersonal reactions when extreme intelligence is recognised; Chapter 5 explores the stereotype of intellectually adept individuals being socially inept; and Chapter 6 looks at how an intensification of such social eccentricity relates to creativity and psychopathology.

Part III – Implications – examines the implications for affected individuals of how extreme intelligence is reacted to. Chapter 7 shows how formative social experiences around intelligence can be enduringly influencing, contributing to the way that suboptimal habits of interaction can become unintentionally perpetuated. Chapter 8 introduces a framework for summarising four main relational styles observed in extremely intelligent individuals. Chapter 9 suggests guidelines on the various issues from the preceding chapters, so as to be able to more often facilitate the better or best of the possible outcomes in different contexts such as parenting and the workplace. It also analyses the change process involved for high-IQ individuals when pursuing better outcomes. The Conclusion draws together the book's central themes and considers what the way we think about and deal with extreme intelligence means for the world around us. Finally, as mentioned above, the Appendix explains the research I carried out that underpins the book.

The Reflective Prompts at the start of each chapter

At the beginning of every chapter focal questions are offered in a shaded box, titled "Reflective Prompt". These probe you as a reader to reflect on your own experiences, feelings, assumptions, and behaviours around extreme intelligence, not as something glamorous and remote that applies only to famous historical figures, but also as something that might manifest – or be hidden – within ordinary everyday life.

These prompts are specifically designed to allow for changes in attitude and opinion over time in accordance with a person's – or a whole culture's – continuing evolution of experience and accumulation of knowledge concerning intelligence. Readers can therefore use these prompts to reflect on changes of this kind that have already taken place during their own lifetimes prior to the point of engaging with this book. Additionally, at the point of finishing the book, readers can go back over the chapters and look at the prompts again to reflect on whether the reading of the book has in itself produced changes in perspective.

These prompts are also ideal for tutors to use interactively with students to create focus and personal involvement experientially during teaching sessions. (As a trainer and supervisor of counsellors and psychotherapists I always incorporate experiential learning methods.) The prompts can also be used, following any such teaching session or series of sessions, as the basis for structuring an assessment of the learning and personal development that has taken place.

Summary

This introduction has explained the Bell Curve of human intelligence. Using a Venn diagram of "potential" overlapping with "performance", it has considered how different intelligence-related terms relate to each other. The importance of intelligence has been acknowledged and its controversy, as different individuals and groups are invested in particular perspectives. It has been asked, how do we *want to* think about extreme intelligence, and why? Challenges in researching intelligence have been introduced, giving examples relating to recruitment of participants and reactions to research findings. The difference between quantitative and qualitative contributions to intelligence research has been explained. The book's unique approach has been identified of integrating insights and knowledge from the fields of intelligence, giftedness, genius, and expertise with those from depth psychology. The book's structure has been outlined, incorporating the social development and predicaments of individuals with very high IQ and the implications for them and the world around us. It has been explained how the book's Reflective Prompts probe readers' personal engagement with the issues involved and provide a teaching resource.

References

American Psychiatric Association. (2013). *Diagnostic and Statistical Manual of Mental Disorders: DSM-5*. (5th ed.). Washington, DC: American Psychiatric Publishing.
British Psychological Society. (2001). *Learning Disability: Definitions and Contexts*. Leicester: British Psychological Society.
Coyle, D. (2010). *The Talent Code – Greatness Isn't Born. It's Grown*. London: Arrow Books.
Favier-Townsend, A. (2014). *Perceived Causes and Long Term Effects of Delayed Academic Achievement in High IQ Adults*. Unpublished PhD thesis, University of Hertfordshire, UK.

Gagné, F. (2013). Yes, giftedness (aka "innate" talent) does exist! In: S. B. Kaufman (Ed.). *The Complexity of Greatness*. Oxford: Oxford University Press. pp. 191–221.

Galton, F. (1869). *Hereditary Genius: An Inquiry into Its Causes and Consequences*. London: Macmillan.

Gladwell, M. (2008). *Outliers: The Story of Success*. London: Allen Lane.

Grobman, J. (2017). *Academic consultation meeting*. [phone call] (Personal communication, 14 January 2017).

Haier, R. J. (2017). *The Neuroscience of Intelligence*. Cambridge: Cambridge University Press.

Hollingworth, L. S. (1926). *Gifted Children: Their Nature and Nurture*. New York: Macmillan.

Intelligence (2014) Special volume: Acquiring expertise: Ability, practice, and other influences. *Intelligence*, 45, (July–August), pp. 1–124.

Meisenberg, G. (2010). The reproduction of intelligence. *Intelligence*, 38, pp. 220–230.

Parkin, E., Kennedy, S., Bate, A., Long, R., Hubble, S. & Powell, A. (2018). *Learning Disability – Policy and Services*. Briefing Paper, Number 07058. London: House of Commons Library.

Silverman, L. K. (2013). *Giftedness 101*. New York: Springer Publishing Company.

Syed, M. (2010). *Bounce: How Champions are Made*. London: Fourth Estate.

PART I
Development

1
MEASURES AND METHODS
The identifying and quantifying of intelligence

> **Reflective Prompt 1:** What has your personal history been in relation to intelligence and IQ? For example, how did you first come across these concepts? How old were you? In what context did this arise? Do you remember what your reaction to this was? What positive or negative associations do you have to these memories? Have your views on intelligence changed over time? How do you feel about the notion of IQ now? Why?

Intelligence is a readily attention-grabbing concept. In the world of advertising, intelligence sells nearly as well as sex: the word "smart" is prefixed as an endorsement to diverse products from sophisticated phones and fridges to investment portfolios and bottled water. But a person needs to be brave to dare to speak or write seriously about intelligence: it is the best studied psychological construct, and also the most controversial (Schneider et al. 2014) – it has even been described as "outrageously controversial" (Plucker & Esping 2014:ix), and "radioactive" (Haier 2017:44), and it has been asserted that "no other concept in science suffers from greater misunderstanding and is plagued with more misconceptions" than the concept of intelligence (Kanazawa 2012:37).

This chapter shows how intelligence as a concept and psychological construct has developed a history and field of enquiry. It introduces methods of measuring intelligence and explains why it is difficult to talk about and has come to be so controversial. The fact of its controversy influences how intelligence as a subject is treated, and how individuals who manifest extreme intelligence are treated. How such individuals are responded to and how this affects them and our wider society is this book's main concern.

The difficulty of talking about intelligence

The Concise Oxford English Dictionary definition of intelligence is "the ability to acquire and apply knowledge and skills" (2011:738). An interest in this kind of ability is recorded from ancient times in several countries – for example, as far back as 2,200 BCE the emperor of China allegedly gave his officials triennial proficiency tests (Kaufman 2009:16). Identifying intelligence in a person is almost invariably presented as a positive, an asset. This is because the ability to acquire and apply knowledge and skills can generally enable a person to navigate whatever situation they might find themselves in as effectively as possible, which is beneficial for themselves and often for those around them. Historically people who became the most prominent contributors to society did so precisely through their acquiring and applying of knowledge and skills, and thereby typically gained rewards in status, influence, and wealth. This positive association extends to intelligence-affiliated terms such as "gifted" which connotes having an advantage, whether this is accurate or true or not. The term "gifted" is thought to derive from the concept of a person being given "gifts from the gods" (Silverman 2013:53).

One of the problems with intelligence being portrayed as a desirable gift rather than it being more neutrally acknowledged as simply one of the many general characteristics that make up an individual, is that it renders intelligence an attribute that a person cannot discuss their own experience of because right from the nursery we are taught not to speak of qualities of our own that could be perceived as positive. This is viewed as boasting – "blowing one's own trumpet" – and frowned upon. And why is there this prohibition?

There is a cross-cultural superstition that an acknowledgment of something being good could make something bad happen. This possibly derives from anticipating, and seeking to avoid inviting, a feared envious attack. In Western society we are raised on fairy tales that early on transmit their warning: in Sleeping Beauty a newborn princess is having gifts bestowed upon her when a wicked fairy swoops in and sentences her to an inevitable wound that is meant to be terminal, but even in its ameliorated form will paralyse her for a century. Similarly, Snow White's beauty attracts dogged attentions bent on nothing less than fatality. Such superstition is widespread in various Middle Eastern and Asian societies where it is encapsulated in the notion of "the evil eye", an omniscient force based in jealousy that can cause serious harm and needs to be defended against. In Hindu society, for example, parents fear that if their newborn baby is admired it could attract the danger of the evil eye, so they protect against this by drawing a black spot or *kala tikka* on the face of the infant to mar its beauty and thereby ward off perilous praise. In Greek tragedy it is hubris that is always followed by nemesis.

When conducting my research interviews, several members of the high-IQ society Mensa spontaneously said that this was a topic one never usually speaks about, and communicated that they were encountering internal resistance against allowing themselves to try to put into words their experiences connected with intelligence. For example, interviewee Tracy made several references to being self-conscious about what she was saying about herself, expressing that she thought it sounded bad: "it sounds so big-headed"; "it sounds so conceited"; "that sounds terrible". Or Helene: "It's a weird thing to talk about, because you don't talk about it often". And Don: "Sorry I feel so arrogant saying I'm intelligent". Although much contemporary advancement has been made in embracing diversity, giving voice to minority experiences, and forbidding discrimination, it is clear in the case of extreme intelligence that this is an area of human diversity that it is still taboo to openly acknowledge and explore even in private conversation.

But it is not only the above reasons that make it difficult to speak about intelligence. Ritchie (2015:2) writes that even mentioning intelligence in "polite company" is greeted as a transgression, because the concept has become associated with elitism, racism, and worse. Kanazawa (2012:1) makes the important point that intelligence is so contentious because it is "somehow" seen as "the most important trait that any human can have", and that there is a tendency to equate intelligence with human worth. He insists strongly (although too simplistically) that intelligence is "just another quantitative trait of an individual like height or weight" (Kanazawa 2012:3). His stated main aim is to break the erroneous equating of intelligence with human worth (Kanazawa 2012:2). This is an aim I fully endorse, although I am critical of Kanazawa's way of trying to achieve it (I say more about this towards the end of the next section). Kanazawa states, surprisingly, that it is "unfathomable" (2012:207) how an equating of intelligence with human worth could ever have come about in the first place. So, how did it come about?

Understanding the controversy

Intelligence being perceived as a quantitative trait means that it is viewed as existing in different levels in different individuals. The positive outcomes mentioned above are associated with higher levels of intelligence. In contrast, various social problems were historically blamed on lower levels of intelligence. We now know from extensive scientific research that higher levels of intelligence are indeed very reliably correlated with higher levels of educational attainment, career achievement, income, health, and longevity, and lower levels of criminality (Hunt 2011; Ritchie 2015; Warne et al. 2018). There are traces as far back as around 380 BCE (in Greek philosopher Plato's *Republic*) (Plucker & Esping 2014:27) of the idea that it would be beneficial if a greater proportion of society could enjoy the positive outcomes associated with higher intelligence. Then in the late 19th and early 20th centuries specific attempts to bring this about started emerging and gathering momentum in ideas and practices that at the time were justified in the most idealistic of terms but which we now look back on as horrific.

It began with scientists and political theorists taking the English naturalist, geologist and biologist Charles Darwin's (Darwin 1859/2012) groundbreaking theory of evolution by natural selection and applying it to people. They began pursuing an agenda of trying to deliberately improve the human species by – instead of leaving such processes to nature – taking it upon themselves to select which human traits they decided were preferable and should be propagated. Darwin's cousin, polymath Francis Galton, in 1883 coined the term "eugenics" by putting together the Greek words *eu* (good) with *genos* (birth) (Plucker & Esping 2014:27). Galton espoused intelligence as a genetically inherited trait that should be promoted and declared its opposite – termed "feeble-mindedness" – as one to eradicate. This was widely accepted: even one of Britain's most admired and cherished statesmen – Winston Churchill – wrote in 1910 in a memo to the prime minister that "[t]he multiplication of the feeble-minded is a very terrible danger to the race" (cited in Brignell 2010). How these traits were then to be identified and differentiated from each other obviously became a major endeavour.

Eugenics movements aimed to steer procreation by means of many practices designed to generate more of what was deemed by various criteria (not only intelligence) to constitute fitter life (termed "positive" eugenics), or to eliminate that which was judged unfit ("negative" eugenics) (Mackintosh 2011). Many countries globally – some much more infamously than others – practiced forms of eugenics. For example, unwanted aspects of humanity were denied entry (the USA's harshest immigration law for over 40 years excluded nationalities that were considered inferior and used intelligence tests to turn thousands away at New York's Ellis Island checkpoint); or segregated, disenfranchised, and oppressed (such as in Apartheid South Africa); or prevented from reproducing through forced sterilisation (widespread in the USA, Canada, Mexico, Japan, Scandinavia, and several East-Central European countries); or even – in Nazi Germany – annihilated through mass extermination (Bashford & Levine 2010; Turda 2017; Okren 2019). Being ruled unfit to live is the utmost accusation possible of having no human worth.

This grim history has spawned extensive backlash. A consequence is that aspects of humanity that were pointed to as reasons for deeming people inferior such as race, sexual orientation, and disability, are now unable to be treated as neutral individual differences. And in the case of intelligence there have even been concerted efforts to deny that individual differences exist at all. This is based on the belief, as Kanazawa (2012:207) puts it, that "everybody is or should be equally intelligent, because everybody is equally worthy as human beings". He explains the logical fallacy in this statement, and he and other authors (Hunt 2011; Ritchie 2015; Haier 2017) argue cogently for the need to distinguish between facts that are discoverable through scientific research – such as individual differences in intelligence – which are in themselves entirely neutral objects of information, and what our reactions are to such facts. Our reactions might be emotional or ideological, such as attaching values to facts, disliking certain facts, or wishing they were instead what we would prefer them to be. Such reactions might provoke us to protest against, conceal, or misrepresent facts. In these ways the straightforward undertaking and disseminating of scientifically rigorous research on intelligence has met with considerable hindrance, including individual researchers being vilified and shunned (see Woodley of Menie et al. 2018). These complications have even resulted in educational institutions opting to cease teaching what has come to be seen as the too-risky subject of intelligence (Woodley of Menie et al. 2018). Warne et al. (2018) undertook an analysis of – where intelligence is still being taught in the USA – what it is that students are being exposed to, by analysing the content of 29 of "the most popular introductory psychology textbooks". They found that 79% of these texts' sections on intelligence research contained inaccurate statements and logical fallacies (which Warne et al. explicate). More about the trajectory of intelligence research is presented in Chapter 2.

The history of the injustices described above creates a pressure to try to rectify them, which can lead to something equally unjust but which is frequently succumbed to – that of practicing discrimination the opposite way around. Where intelligence is concerned, 21st-century discrimination against intelligence – or "anti-intellectualism" – can often be noticed. One quick example is that in the same book in which Kanazawa (2012) advocates strongly for sound logic and value-free scientific reasoning to prevail, he throughout insensitively pokes humorously framed insults at extremely intelligent individuals. He freely calls them "incompetent", "stupid", and "life's ultimate losers", in a manner that would almost certainly have been unpublishable had the individuals he was writing about been identified as having a disability rather than high ability. Kanazawa unfortunately goes about his aim of trying to break the equating of intelligence with human worth by mocking highly intelligent individuals as not really having much worth.

So far we have been working with a simple dictionary definition of what intelligence is, but the academic literature provides much greater complexity.

The academic literature's definitions and theories of intelligence

Plucker & Esping (2014:16–20) fill five full pages with definitions of intelligence from 19 different learned sources. Something that all of these have in common is that intelligence is seen as an ability or skill, usually defined as a trait (a characteristic of the individual that is reasonably stable over time and that is revealed in many situations) (Hunt 2011:12) that is mental or cognitive in nature. With this, as explained in the Introduction, we run into the difference between observable performance (such as a person's adeptness at processing information) and the underlying trait which is theorised to be powering this performance.

18   Development

Figure 1.1 depicts – with the permission of Professor Jonathan Plucker, Johns Hopkins University – his summary of what is to date already an extensive history of attempts to define, understand, and measure human intelligence.

An interactive version of this map is available at www.intelltheory.com/map.shtml. I will present very briefly here, in chronological order of their development, four prominent theories of intelligence that provide the most useful reference points for the current book's purposes. The first two have proven important to intelligence researchers, underpinning substantial ongoing theorising about, researching of, and measuring of intelligence. They are psychometric theories because they are concerned with what components underlie performances on intelligence tests. The second two do not have the same empirical support or significance for academic research but are distinctive for their widespread popular appeal and sociocultural impact. They move away from a focus on test-taking to incorporate other behaviours in wider contexts.

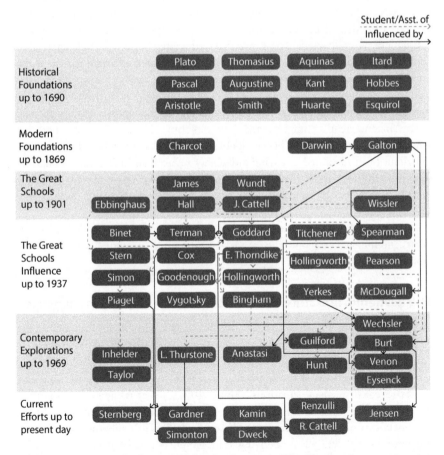

FIGURE 1.1   History of influences in the development of intelligence theory and testing

Spearman's g

This is one of the oldest modern theories of intelligence and has turned out to also be the most important and enduring one for which there is the greatest support in significant bodies of empirical evidence. Introduced by Charles Spearman (1904), *g* stands for the general factor of intelligence. He devised the statistical technique of factor analysis – still today the favoured procedure for analysing the structure of human abilities (Mackintosh 2011) – through which he showed that scores on all mental tests were positively correlated. He termed this "positive manifold" (cited in Ritchie 2015). From this Spearman concluded that it was a single core capability or power, which he called *g*, that gave rise to all cognitive abilities. He termed the specific skills (such as mathematical or spatial) that particular tests or sub-tests measure "s-factors" (cited in Ritchie 2015). More recent models of intelligence (see Warne et al. 2018), such as CHC theory, are still based on accepting the existence of *g*, but they theorise different ways in which *g* as a general ability relates to other "midlevel" or broad abilities as well as to more specific or narrow abilities; how many of these different abilities there are; and whether and how they are all related hierarchically to each other.

The Cattell–Horn theory of fluid and crystallised intelligences

Raymond Bernard Cattell was a student of Spearman, and Cattell and his own most famous student John Horn (Horn & Cattell 1966) distinguished between fluid and crystallised intelligence. Fluid intelligence, represented as *Gf*, is what responds to novel stimuli and solves new problems through active analysing, reasoning and processing, and encoding short-term memories. Crystallised intelligence, or *Gc*, is the accumulation and application of learned skills and facts. Physiological efficiency such as speed of reaction increases *Gf*, and education that builds knowledge retention increases *Gc*. The distinction between these two different kinds of intelligence has proven very useful for almost all subsequent theorising about and measuring of intelligence. CHC theory, mentioned above, stands for "Cattell–Horn–Carroll", and involves an amalgamation of the original Cattell–Horn theory with later work by John Carroll (Mackintosh 2011; Plucker & Esping 2014).

Gardner's multiple intelligences

Howard Gardner (1983) sought to extend the collection of competencies traditionally associated with intelligence beyond the cognitive domain to other behaviours including physical, social, and spiritual, and named these as additional kinds of intelligence. He theorised that there are several separate powers of problem solving and creativity that each relate to different domains of human experience and activity, and after his initial naming of these he added to them so that eventually he had nine different so-called multiple intelligences:

linguistic, logical/mathematical, spatial, bodily-kinaesthetic, musical, interpersonal, intrapersonal, naturalist, and spiritual (Gardner 2011). This conceptualisation has been very popular but remains unsubstantiated by empirical evidence (Waterhouse 2006; Hunt 2011; Ritchie 2015; Warne et al. 2018). Its popularity relates to the way it plays into the already-established cultural value of intelligence as something important, but provides a language for what intelligence is that shifts it away from its accumulated negative associations with exclusivity and rejection on the basis of cognitive capability. Instead it introduces inclusivity and acceptance whereby many different and non-cognitive capabilities are newly esteemed as forms of intelligence.

Sternberg's theory of successful intelligence

Robert Sternberg's theory of successful intelligence (1997; 1999) supersedes a theory he previously became known for, called his triarchic theory of intelligence (1984; 1985). The triarchic theory, as its title suggests, identified three aspects of intelligence in terms of how they contributed to a person being able to get on well in "the real world" (Sternberg 1984:271). It appears that Sternberg considered he would himself get on better in that "real world" by making his work more accessible to non-specialist audiences, and accordingly evolved his theory into something more catchily named and more simply explained. He defines successful intelligence as "the ability to achieve success in life, given one's personal standards, within one's sociocultural context" (Sternberg 1999:293). The processing skills he identifies as contributing to this are still three in number, named as analytical, creative, and practical. He explains that achieving this kind of success involves a person being able to adapt to, shape, and select environments, and also capitalise on his or her strengths and correct and compensate for weaknesses.

This section has focused on the identifying of intelligence, and now we turn to the issue of quantifying intelligence.

Is there ever any good reason to try to measure intelligence?

At the beginning of the 20th century the French education ministry grappled with what to do about children who were not thriving in France's prevailing system of schooling. Psychologist Alfred Binet was commissioned to devise an assessment method for matching children with educational programmes suited to their capabilities (Hunt 2011). The tests Binet and colleagues created became the first successful modern intelligence tests. Professor Lewis Terman at Stanford University translated the tests into English and modified them, resulting in the Stanford-Binet Intelligence Test which is still in use today in regularly updated forms. It was a version of this originally devised intelligence test that was used by the USA to accept or reject potential immigrants (Plucker & Esping 2014).

The previous paragraph highlights two historical rationales for measuring intelligence: one centres on how to match individuals with programmes (educational, or occupational) to which their capabilities are best suited, and the other centres on whether individuals are being accepted or rejected. Proponents of testing highlight the usefulness of the former, whilst detractors criticise the discriminatory effects of the latter. The "matching" rationale inevitably also relates to acceptance/rejection, because being matched entails being accepted onto a programme that has been determined to be suitable and/or rejected from one deemed unsuitable. As Chapter 3 will emphasise, we all dread rejection. People can easily conflate having their capabilities judged as not being appropriate for a particular programme or role with being judged unacceptable as human beings, and how test results are communicated and handled can strongly influence this conflation (a conflation which was of course also devastatingly fuelled by eugenics). Any test associated with a possible outcome of rejection is not going to be popular. And depending on what is at stake – life in a chosen country, a coveted career, or even, historically, the right to stay alive – the significance of a rejection can be and often has been profound.

However, there are important pragmatic uses of intelligence testing. It is such testing that can determine the competencies a person has following a serious head injury, or that can determine whether children need specialised education or elderly persons are able to manage their own affairs, or whether criminals have the mental capacity to be held responsible for their crimes. Intelligence testing also provides, as Hunt (2011) explains, the most efficient and democratic way we currently have of dealing with the necessity of assigning people to required roles in large societies. For example, when staffing a country's military, for which tens of thousands of soldiers are needed for diverse roles of varying complexity, testing allows anyone to apply and assists recruiters to assign applicants to appropriate roles. Also, providing education or training is costly and testing helps identify which are the best candidates in which to invest such limited resources based on their likelihood of proceeding to work effectively in the role for which they are given preparation. Intelligence testing is still the most reliable large-scale predictor we currently have of job performance (Haier 2017). How, then, do such tests work?

Can intelligence actually be measured?

In taking up the commission mentioned above, Binet (1903) noticed that normally developing children could master increasingly complex intellectual tasks as they got older. He devised test questions to target the different intellectual levels ordinarily expected at different ages. He could then see by which tasks any child taking the test could master whether they were functioning at a mental age that matched their chronological age or at a mental age usually expected of a younger or older child. He derived a numerical value for the child's level of functioning by dividing their mental age by their chronological age and multiplying by 100. He did not call this an IQ score. At around the same time the concept of Intelligence Quotient as a measure of human intelligence was originated by German psychologist William Stern (Lamiell 1996), and it was first abbreviated to IQ by Terman (Ritchie 2015).

All subsequent IQ tests share with this original method the similarity that they involve someone deciding what constitutes appropriate intellectual tasks to include in the test, setting such tasks at differing levels of complexity, and creating a formula – a statistical calculation – that records how any test-taker performs on those tasks in relation to the performances of other test-takers (see information about IQ scoring and the Bell Curve in the Introduction). A main problem with this is that there is no ratio scale measure for intelligence such as the measuring of height in metres or liquid in litres (Haier 2017). I will list below four main points about IQ tests:

1. *There is a substantial overlap in how all IQ tests work as well as other assessment methods that are similar but not named as IQ tests.* Although the use of forms of testing is widespread for selection to schools, universities, and jobs, these are not usually called intelligence tests. However, the way they work is highly correlated with tests that are called intelligence tests. IQ tests measure abstract thinking, involving different aspects of or combinations of reasoning (inductive and deductive), spatial ability (sometimes termed visual–spatial reasoning), memory, processing speed, and knowledge (Ritchie 2015). Reasoning can be assessed by matrix tasks (choosing the correct picture that completes a given sequence by finding the rule that governs that sequence), or by verbal or numerical tasks. Measures of spatial ability involve tasks such as having to mentally rotate a given image. Tasks involving memory assess working memory, i.e. they assess how much of a given set of information a person can hold in mind and then repeat back, use for solving a complex problem, or answer questions on later. Measures of speed include how quickly a person can complete a task or how fast his or her reaction time is. Knowledge is assessed in tasks relating to vocabulary and general knowledge questions. Some tests measure one or another of these main areas (e.g. Raven's Progressive Matrices which measures only non-verbal reasoning ability), and some measure more than one or all of them (e.g. the different revisions of the Wechsler Adult Intelligence Scale, or WAIS, measures all of them). It is usual that if a person is good at one aspect on a test they are also good at the others. However, some tests give a breakdown of verbal IQ (tasks involving words) versus performance IQ (tasks involving pictures, digits, or symbols), and some people can have discrepancies between these scores (more is said about this in Chapters 5 and 6). Group differences can also be apparent: for example, whilst there is no difference between males and females in general intelligence (Johnson et al. 2008), in terms of specific abilities males tend to score higher on spatial ability and females higher on verbal measures (Miller & Halpern 2014).

2. *IQ tests differ from each other according to the particular purpose they have been designed to serve.* For example, it is essential to assess visual–spatial competence in would-be aviators, but this is irrelevant for potential lawyers. SAT tests in the USA are routinely administered to university applicants to predict whether they will succeed at completing a course (Hunt 2011). The most widely used tests that are individually administered by a trained professional are the regularly updated WAIS and the WISC (the Wechsler Intelligence Scale for Children), originally designed in the late 1930s by psychologist David Wechsler (Hunt 2011). Individually administered tests include much more extensive tasks of different kinds (Kaufman 2009) than do group-administered tests which can test large numbers of candidates simultaneously. Group tests were first designed during the First World War by Harvard psychologist Robert Yerkes who designed the Army Alpha test to assess new US military recruits (Ritchie 2015). The contemporary version is the Armed Services Vocational Aptitude Battery (ASVAB). This test requires lower language skill than the SAT does because it is considered that soldiers can succeed without the level of language skill that a university candidate would need to succeed (Hunt 2011). In the UK the current (since 2018) equivalent is the British Army Selection Test.
3. *There is very high correlation between results in all IQ tests.* Even one very short single-format test just measuring verbal ability (e.g. a three-minute test designed by British psychologist Alan Baddeley) gives results that are similar to extensive batteries of sub-tests (Hunt 2011), and the results of even seemingly unrelated tests always correlate with each other. This has been proven in studies of over 460 sets of intelligence testing data (Carroll 1993). This positive manifold is one of the most well-replicated findings in psychological science (Ritchie 2015). It is what endorses the idea of Spearman's *g*, that there is a general ability that underlies all manifestations of different specific abilities.
4. *IQ tests are imperfect and there will always be exceptions to their predictive accuracy, however they generally serve effectively a necessary purpose in educational, occupational, medical, and legal settings for which no better substitute has yet been found.* IQ tests assess people only at one point in time in a manner that is abstract and out of context with anything else in their lives, and cannot reflect capabilities such as longer-term persistence in sticking with a problem (Hunt 2011). In some instances this will compromise the accuracy of the result. An example is that written IQ tests will disadvantage dyslexic test-takers. The presence of dyslexia or any other psychological or developmental condition can mask a person's true ability, and when this is the case with a person who has high ability or giftedness it is termed twice exceptionality or 2e for short (see Ronksley-Pavia 2015), or dual and multiple exceptionality (DME) (Montgomery 2015). Steele (1997) showed that when racial, socioeconomic, gender, and age groups are negatively stereotyped as being unsuccessful academically, this could undermine the performance of individuals from such groups because of their fear of being associated with that negative stereotype. However, this phenomenon,

termed "stereotype threat" (Steele 1997:614), does not alone account for differences in test scores in different groups (Sackett et al. 2004; Warne et al. 2018). Test scores have been shown to predict academic success irrespective of socioeconomic status (SES), age, sex, race, and other variables (Haier 2017:18). Probably the most common criticism is the claim that IQ tests are culturally biased and advantage test-takers who are familiar with the knowledge base that test-makers are drawing on. It is ironic that one of the original reasons for using testing was to assess a person's capability separately from what educational benefits he or she might have had (Hunt 2011). Remembering Cattell-Horn's distinction between *Gf* and *Gc*, it is only *Gc* that relates to acculturation and previous education. It can be difficult to separate elements of a test from being influenced by *Gc*, however, tests have been designed that do almost exclusively measure *Gf*, the most well-known and effective of these being Raven's Progressive Matrices (Kanazawa 2012). Haier (2017) explains that a test is only biased if its scores consistently over- or underpredict performance, and that this is not the case with IQ tests, although there will always be exceptions to the evidenced general trend. Work on testing methods is ongoing so as to make these as fair as possible. Overall, however, IQ tests have proven for over a century to have generally high validity and reliability (Kaufman 2009; Kanazawa 2012; Haier 2017).

Everything described above relates to the psychometric approach to quantifying intelligence, where the taking of a test produces an IQ score. Recent progress in neuroimaging has shown that IQ test scores are correlated to a variety of structural and functional measures of the brain (Haier 2017). For example, echoing the male versus female strengths shown in IQ test results as reported above, it has been found that there is more grey matter in male brains in posterior regions related to visual-spatial processing and more grey matter in female brains in the frontal lobes related to language (Haier 2017:88). With further advancements in identifying physiological aspects of intelligence it might eventually become possible to measure intelligence not by administering an IQ test, but by interpreting images of a person's brain, or running a DNA test (Haier 2017). Another possible alternative way of measuring intelligence that is being researched is "chronometrics" (Haier 2017:168). This involves measuring the speed of information processing in the brain in units of milliseconds, which might be able to provide a quantitative assessment of intelligence on a ratio scale.

However, returning to IQ scores, as explained in the Introduction, an IQ score of 130 and above constitutes extreme intelligence. How does this relate to what we would call genius?

Quantifying genius

In terms of IQ scores, the figure of 140 and above was in 1925 proposed by Terman as constituting genius (cited in Simonton 2009:21). The Oxford

Concise Dictionary definition of genius is "exceptional intellectual or creative power or other natural ability", and "an exceptionally intelligent or able person" (2011:594). We usually think of a genius as someone who has proven their exceptional abilities through exceptional achievement, and these are often people who are no longer living – such as Shakespeare or Einstein – who we evaluate retrospectively in accordance with the longevity and continuing impact of their work. Measuring the genius of such persons has been attempted with "historiometric" methods (Simonton 2007).

Historiometrics involves gathering biographical and historical information then quantifying it and subjecting it to statistical analysis. Attempts have even been made to assign IQ scores to historically prominent achievers. Terman (1917) did this by adopting the formula that Binet had first employed for assessing children's mental versus chronological ages. Using biographical information about Francis Galton that stated that he could, for example, read at the age of two-and-a-half, Terman calculated that Galton's IQ would have been close to 200. Other historiometric methods have involved rating prominent historical figures according to their ultimate influence; ranking such individuals according to the amount of space allocated to each in biographical dictionaries and encyclopaedias; or surveying experts on their nominations of and ratings of candidates (Simonton 2007). For achievers in science, the number of citations their work receives is used as a measure of their impact, and for composers of classical music, the number of times their work is recorded or performed (Simonton 2007). Using multiple different measures reduces subjective bias and increases the validity of the results. For example, by a combination of space measures, expert surveys, and performance frequency, the three top composers are almost invariably placed – albeit not always in the same order – as Beethoven, Mozart, and J. S. Bach (Simonton 2007).

Moving away from formal attempts to identify and quantify intelligence, what is more to the point for my concerns in this book is a consideration of how intelligence manifests in everyday life and how people in general social situations handle the phenomenon of intelligence.

Identifying extreme intelligence and intelligence generally in everyday life

Typical characteristics associated with extreme intelligence are discussed in Chapter 3's section "Person: the extremely high-IQ individual". Such characteristics and how they manifest are further explored throughout the rest of the book. What can be said here, though, is that different bands of IQ score have repeatedly been shown to correlate with different general life outcomes. For example, IQ scores have been shown to accurately predict who will get the highest exam results, who will stay at school for longer, and who will be more likely to go on to get degrees and other qualifications (Ritchie 2015). Higher IQ is correlated with higher educational qualifications, which in turn are correlated with higher income. Using data from the US Bureau of Labor Statistics, Hunt (2011:326) shows that median weekly earnings are directly proportionate to level of educational qualification: at the bottom of the scale, individuals with no high school diploma averaged $400 per week, and at the top of the scale, individuals with doctoral degrees averaged nearly $1600 per week. Mackintosh (2011:198) presents data on IQ scores in relation to occupation. This shows, at the bottom end of the spectrum, that the mean IQ for miners is 91, and at the top, that the mean IQ for engineers, lawyers, and accountants is 127–128.

This top measure of 127–128 still falls short, however, of our definition of extreme intelligence. These figures do not, therefore, tell us anything helpful about extreme intelligence in particular. Similarly, Herrnstein & Murray's (1994) classification system of "cognitive classes", repeated in Kanazawa (2012:54), places its top IQ band at "IQ > 125", termed "very bright". This makes no distinction between the capacities and experiences of individuals who, although all within that top band, can still be whole standard deviations apart from each other. One thing that is apparent in a lot of this data, is that it is the scores at the top of the average range of intelligence that are most often associated with successes of the above-cited everyday-life kinds. What sorts of outcomes are associated specifically with IQ in the range of extreme intelligence, and whether such a level of intelligence is a benefit or a liability, is examined in Chapter 6.

In ordinary daily life people do appraise each other according to how intelligent they are perceived as being. People can by appearance and subtle behaviour cues assess a stranger's measured intelligence more accurately than expected by chance (Murphy et al. 2003; Lee et al. 2017), and people regularly react to negative violations of behaviour expectations by calling the actions involved "stupid" (Aczel et al. 2015). People are usually described as intelligent when they are perceived to be behaving in a manner that the viewer regards as capable and values. There are five points related to this that I want to emphasise, and these also act as an overview of what I think is important to take away from this chapter.

1. *An appraisal of intelligence rests on a perception.* This means that what is perceived might be different from what a person's capability actually is. There might be a capability present that is not being perceived, either because it is being somehow constrained or because a demonstration of it is being voluntarily withheld. An example of the former is Tolan's (1996) well-known critique of identifying giftedness by achievement. She used the analogy of a cheetah in a cage: the cheetah has the capability to run very fast, but this is not perceived because of the circumstantial constraint of it being in a cage. Constraints to the expression or realisation of high ability can come in many forms, through external barriers such as lack of opportunity (including that caused by gender or race discrimination) or internal barriers such as the difficulties and/or disabilities of dual and multiple exceptionality,

or stereotype threat. When demonstration of a capability is voluntarily withheld, this often relates to motivation. This is articulated by Hunt's (2011) crucial distinction between "can do" and "will do": if the cheetah is unconstrained – for example, it is in a wide open plain rather than in a cage and has no condition holding it back – just because it can run does not mean that it will. It will run when it identifies a worthwhile reason to run – i.e. it has the motivation to run – and also when it judges that it is safe to run.

2. *Any appraisal of intelligence is always relative.* The whole method of obtaining IQ scores is relative, i.e. results are measured relative to others who take the test. Socially, the appraisal of intelligence is also relative. If a person is performing at a level more capable and impressive than the observer is accustomed to seeing, then that person will be described as intelligent. If the person is performing at a level lower than what the observer is accustomed to, it will be the reverse. The Fang, a society of mixed agriculturalists and hunters in Equatorial Guinea, define intelligent people as those "who do not get lost in the forest" (Hunt 2011:21). People living in urban environments in complex post-industrial societies who perhaps never go near a forest would be likely to describe as intelligent someone who shows proficiency in operating sophisticated modern technologies. However, the underlying mental capacities that produce these functions that are differently esteemed in different cultures – spatial orientation in a forest, or capable application of learning about a new computer's functionality – are the same ones that are assessed in abstraction in IQ tests.

3. *Intelligence is understood to be a trait, i.e. something someone "has".* In the analogy in No. 1 above, the capability of running is seen to be possessed by the cheetah. Similarly, intelligence is assumed to be possessed by a person. It is not considered that manifestation of intelligence in one context or set of circumstances rather than another means that it is the context or circumstance that is producing the intelligence. It is considered that the intelligence is a trait that the presiding circumstances are facilitating – or masking – the detection of. For example, once motor neurone disease rendered Stephen Hawking paralysed and unable to speak, without the provision of a computer to facilitate his communication no-one would have been able to detect his extreme intelligence. However, when a computer made communication possible, the intelligence that was manifest was seen as a trait existing within Hawking, not as residing in or being created by the computer.

4. *A capability is only labelled intelligent if it is esteemed.* A person could be seen to be gargling very capably, but this behaviour is not valued so it is not judged intelligent. This point, and the one in No. 2 above, relates to Sternberg's and Gardner's definitions of intelligence as something that is judged within its sociocultural context. The problem with this is that if others do not understand a person's behaviour, it will not be valued, but this does not necessarily mean it is not intelligent. There are many examples of individuals

whose genius only came to be recognised and valued posthumously. A famous example in art is Vincent van Gogh, who by the time of his death in 1890 had only sold one painting (Naifeh & Smith 2012). And an example in science is Gregor Johann Mendel, now hailed as the founder of genetics, whose work was ignored and only came to be understood many years after his death in 1884 (Klein & Klein 2011).

5. *An appraisal of intelligence is not neutral.* The fact of intelligence constituting a trait that is valued means that describing someone as intelligent is a positive, usually used as a compliment. Describing someone as unintelligent is a negative, often used as an insult. Someone being called an "imbecile" or "idiot" – which incidentally were original French terms for actual specified categories of lower intelligence used by Binet (Nicolas et al. 2013) – is an expression of frustration with that person, denoting an experience of not managing to "get through to" (be understood by) them, finding they are "taking too long", or doing something "the wrong way". Something being done well or better or faster than expected is labelled intelligent. But, as in the example of Mendel above, we might judge behaviour as unintelligent because we do not understand it: someone might not be doing something in the way that you expect because they have superior intelligence and are using a method that you do not (yet) understand, or you might not be "getting through" to them because you are not explaining yourself clearly enough.

These points relate to colloquial thinking about intelligence, but they are also relevant to the professional field of theorising and researching intelligence.

Summary

This chapter has introduced the difficulty of talking about intelligence and explained its controversy. The defining of intelligence – both academically and colloquially – has been discussed, as well as ways of measuring it. Four main points made about IQ tests are that there is substantial overlap in how they all work; they differ according to their purpose; there is high correlation between results in all IQ tests; and although they are imperfect they serve effectively a necessary purpose. It has been argued that – in ordinary life as well as in the evaluation of intelligence in professional contexts – an appraisal of intelligence rests on a perception which is always relative and might or might not be accurate; that intelligence is understood to be a trait; that a capability is only labelled intelligent if it is esteemed; and therefore that an appraisal of intelligence is not neutral. The controversy and non-neutrality surrounding intelligence, and the fact that a lot of data we have on intelligence does not distinguish the range that comprises extreme intelligence, affects how individuals who manifest extreme intelligence are understood and treated. Therefore, beyond these issues of identifying and quantifying intelligence is the question of how persons with extreme intelligence – and those around them – experience this and live with this. This is this book's main concern, and this will be engaged with fully after the next chapter which first addresses what the causes are of extreme intelligence.

References

Aczel, B., Palfi, B. & Kekecs, Z. (2015). What is stupid? People's conception of unintelligent behaviour. *Intelligence*, 53, pp. 51–58.
Bashford, A. & Levine, P. (2010). *The Oxford Handbook of the History of Eugenics*. New York: Oxford University Press.
Binet, A. (1903). *L'Etude expérimentale de l'intelligence*. Reprint 2004 s.l. Paris: L'Harmattan.
Brignell, V. (2010). British eugenics disabled. *The New Statesman*. [online] Available at: www.newstatesman.com/society/2010/12/british-eugenics-disabled. [Accessed 16 October 2018].
Carroll, J. B. (1993). *Human Cognitive Abilities: A Survey of Factor-Analytic Studies*. Cambridge: Cambridge University Press.
The Concise Oxford English Dictionary. (2011). Oxford: Oxford University Press.
Darwin, C. (1859/2012). *On the Origin of the Species by Means of Natural Selection*. London: Arcturus Publishing Ltd.
Galton, F. (1883). *Inquiries into Human Faculty and Its Development*. London: Macmillan.
Gardner, H. (1983). *Frames of Mind: The Theory of Multiple Intelligences*. New York: Basic Books.
Gardner, H. (2011). *Frames of Mind – The Theory of Multiple Intelligences*. New York: Basic Books.
Haier, R. J. (2017). *The Neuroscience of Intelligence*. Cambridge: Cambridge University Press.
Herrnstein, R. J. & Murray, C. (1994). *The Bell Curve: Intelligence and Class Structure in American Life*. New York: Free Press.
Horn, J. L. & Cattell, R. B. (1966). Refinement and test of the theory of fluid and crystallised general intelligences. *Journal of Educational Psychology*, 57(5), pp. 253–270.
Hunt, E. (2011). *Human Intelligence*. New York: Cambridge University Press.
Johnson, W., Carothers, A. & Deary, I. J. (2008). Sex differences in variability in general intelligence: a new look at the old question. *Perspectives on Psychological Science*, 3(6), pp. 518–531.
Kanazawa, S. (2012). *The Intelligence Paradox*. Hoboken, NJ: John Wiley & Sons.
Kaufman, A. S. (2009). *IQ Testing 101*. New York: Springer Publishing Company.
Klein, J. & Klein, N. (2011). *Solitude of a Humble Genius – Gregor Johann Mendel: Volume 1: Formative Years*. Berlin: Springer Publishing Company .
Lamiell, J. T. (1996). William Stern: More than "the IQ guy". In: G. A. Kimble; C. A. Boneau & M. Wertheimer (Eds.). *Portraits of Pioneers in Psychology*, Vol. II. Hillsdale, NJ: Erlbaum. pp. 73–85.
Lee, A. J., Hibbs, C., Wright, M. J., Martin, N. G., Keller, M. C. & Zietsch, B. P. (2017). Assessing the accuracy of perceptions of intelligence based on heritable facial features. *Intelligence*, 64, pp. 1–8.
Mackintosh, N. J. (2011). *IQ and Human Intelligence*. (2nd ed.). Oxford: Oxford University Press.
Miller, D. I. & Halpern, D. F. (2014). The new science of cognitive sex differences. *Trends in Cognitive Sciences*, 18(1), pp. 37–45.

Montgomery, D. (2015). *Teaching Gifted Children with Special Educational Needs*. London: Routledge.
Murphy, N. A., Hall, J. A. & Colvin, C. R. (2003). Accurate intelligence assessments in social interactions: mediators and gender effects. *Journal of Personality*, 71(3), pp. 465–493.
Naifeh, S. & Smith, G. W. (2012). *Van Gogh – The Life*. London: Profile Books.
Nicolas, S., Andrieu, B., Croizet, J.-C., Sanitioso, R. B. & Burman, J. T. (2013). Sick? Or slow? On the origins of intelligence as a psychological object. *Intelligence*, 41(5), pp. 699–711.
Okren, D. (2019). *The Guarded Gate*. New York: Scribner.
Plucker, J. A. & Esping, A. (2014). *Intelligence 101*. New York: Springer Publishing Company.
Ritchie, S. J. (2015). *Intelligence – All That Matters*. London: John Murray Learning.
Ronksley-Pavia, M. (2015). A model of twice-exceptionality: explaining and defining the apparent paradoxical combination of disability and giftedness in childhood. *Journal for the Education of the Gifted*, 38(3), pp. 318–340.
Sackett, P. R., Hardison, C. M. & Cullen, M. J. (2004). On the value of correcting mischaracterizations of stereotype threat research. *American Psychologist*, 59(1), pp. 48–49.
Schneider, W., Niklas, F. & Schmiedeler, S. (2014). Intellectual development from early childhood to early adulthood: the impact of early IQ differences on stability and change over time. *Learning and Individual Differences*, 32, pp. 156–162.
Silverman, L. K. (2013). *Giftedness 101*. New York: Springer Publishing Company.
Simonton, D. K. (2007). Historiometrics. In: N. J. Salkind (Ed.). *Encyclopedia of Measurement and Statistics*, Vol. 2. Thousand Oaks, CA: Sage. p. 441.
Simonton, D. K. (2009). *Genius 101*. New York: Springer Publishing Company.
Spearman, C. (1904). "General intelligence," objectively determined and measured. *American Journal of Psychology*, 15, pp. 201–293.
Steele, C. M. (1997). A threat in the air: how stereotypes shape intellectual identity and performance. *American Psychologist*, 52(6), pp. 613–629.
Sternberg, R. J. (1984). Toward a triarchic theory of human intelligence. *Behavioral and Brain Sciences*, 7, pp. 269–287.
Sternberg, R. J. (1985). *Beyond IQ: A Triarchic Theory of Human Intelligence*. New York: Cambridge University Press.
Sternberg, R. J. (1997). *Successful Intelligence*. New York: Plume.
Sternberg, R. J. (1999). The theory of successful intelligence. *Review of General Psychology*, 3, pp. 292–316.
Terman, L. M. (1917). The intelligence quotient of Francis Galton in childhood. *American Journal of Psychology*, 28, pp. 209–215.
Tolan, S. S. (1996). *Is It a Cheetah?* [online] Available at: www.stephanietolan.com/is_it_a_cheetah.htm. [Accessed 11 September 2016].
Turda, M. (Ed.) (2017). *The History of East-Central European Eugenics, 1900–1945: Sources and Commentaries*. London: Bloomsbury.
Warne, R. T., Astle, M. C. & Hill, J. C. (2018). What do undergraduates learn about human intelligence? An analysis of introductory psychology textbooks. *Archives of Scientific Psychology*, 6, pp. 32–50.
Waterhouse, L. (2006). Multiple intelligences, the Mozart effect, and emotional intelligence: a critical review. *Educational Psychologist*, 41(4), pp. 207–225.
Woodley of Menie, M. A., Dutton, E., Figueredo, A.-J., Carl, N., Debes, F., Hertler, S., Irwing, P., Kura, K., Lynn, R., Madison, G., Meisenber, G., Miller, E. M., te Nijenhuis, J., Nyborg, H. & Rindermann, H. (2018). Communicating intelligence research: media misrepresentation, the Gould Effect, and unexpected forces. *Intelligence*, 70, pp. 84–87.

2
THE ROOTS OF DIFFERENCE

How is it that some people stand out so much from others?

> **Reflective Prompt 2:** Can you recall an occasion when someone stood out to you for achieving something that you didn't expect was possible, which you found astonishing and impressive? Describe what made his or her achievement unexpected, and what made it impressive. What was your explanation then of what made it possible for this person to achieve that? Do you know what caused you to rely on that particular explanation rather than on an alternative explanation? What would your explanation now be?

Having outlined the defining and measuring of intelligence, we now turn to the question of what it is that produces the highest measured extremes in intelligence and how this relates to observed cases of exceptional performance: what is it that makes someone stand out so much from others? In one of classicist Caroline Lawrence's historical novels based in Ancient Rome she explores proficiency as well as the taboo against a person asserting his or her own prowess. At one point her character Flavia Gemina disconcertedly glances around before addressing the physician Titus Flavius Cosmus:

> "I'm not being impolite, but isn't it hubris," she whispered, "to say you're the best?"

He replies:

> It's not hubris. It's the truth. Thanks to the five principles of Asclepiades and my skilled fingers and especially my nose, I am the best!
>
> *(Lawrence 2003:82)*

In Cosmus's reply are the exact factors that can be – and extensively have been – scrutinised when questioning what it is that produces exceptional performance: is it primarily the accumulation of knowledge (this physician had studied Asclepiades), or extensive practise that has brought about mastery (the skill his fingers have acquired), or is it something innate in the person's particular individual biological make-up (in this case his unique sensitivity in discerning smells – i.e. his nose)? And if a combination of all of these, in what proportions? The current chapter first explains the main debate pertinent to this, then looks at how this relates to the trajectory of intelligence research, before ending with an analogy that encapsulates the main issues involved.

The nature versus nurture debate

It is one of the earliest studies of genius, by Francis Galton in 1874, that gave us in its title the phrase "nature and nurture" which has since become so ubiquitous. Galton was fascinated by people who stood out significantly from others in their accomplishments, and he saw this as being brought about by their intelligence. He became convinced that intelligence was genetically inherited because he traced that many high achievements were concentrated across several generations of certain family lineages whereas other families did not produce any notable offspring (Galton 1869). (A more recent example of this is that since the introduction of Nobel Prizes in 1901, in the science categories of this extremely rare and prestigious award there have been eight cases where a winner had a son or daughter who also became a winner, and a case of two brothers both winning – Nobel Laureates Facts n.d.). The interpretation – whether correct or not – that such a trend is genetic, is what constitutes the "nature", or biologically determinist, view of ability. It is this view that dominated the era of eugenics. It is also what informed educational policies that were based on selection according to ability, such as the system instated by the UK's Education Act 1944 which lasted through to the early 1970s. This involved using "11-plus" assessments – highly correlated with IQ tests – on all junior school children to determine which kind of senior school they would attend. In effect this would mean either an academically demanding and ambitious school (called "grammar" schools), or a school focused on more practical skills and not supportive of entry to higher education ("secondary modern" schools). There are two crucial questions here, which relate to Galton's two assumptions: firstly, is intelligence implicated in performance (with higher intelligence leading to higher performance); and secondly, is level of intelligence innate (genetically determined)?

A strong denial that intelligence is innate came at around the time that the above-mentioned educational policy was ending, with Leon Kamin's (1974) *The Science and Politics of IQ*. This "nurture" position highlights the role of environmental influences in constructing and then reinforcing observed differences in performance. The disagreement between the nature and the nurture proponents is intense. Two prominent books showing this opposition are Stephen Jay

Gould's *The Mismeasure of Man* (1981) (nurture) and Richard Herrnstein & Charles Murray's (1994) infamous *The Bell Curve* (nature). Arguments are put forward with at times ardent and emotive language (e.g. Shenk 2010), sometimes accusing their opponents of scholarly misconduct such as the misrepresenting of research findings – see the debate between Gagné (nature) and Ericsson (nurture) in Kaufman (2013). Gagné (2013:192) asserted "nature" as the mainstream position and "nurture" as being represented by only "a small minority of researchers", namely Howe et al. (1998) in the UK and Ericsson et al. (2007) in the USA. Even if it is true that Anders Ericsson was in a minority, his prolific work (e.g. Ericsson et al. 1993; 2007; 2018) has had very wide impact.

Practise and expertise

Ericsson argued that observable exceptional performance – which he termed "expertise" – had no biological basis but was developed exclusively through long-term careful cultivation, which he measured as requiring 10,000 hours of what he explicated as "deliberate practise". This message was repeated over and over again in a spate of popular books published between 2008 and 2014 (including Colvin 2008; Coyle 2010; Shenk 2010; Syed 2010; Stobart 2014), probably the most well-known one being Malcolm Gladwell's (2008) *Outliers*. These books often rehash the same data, such as a story from Ericsson's research on memory involving an undergraduate student who perfected the fast memorisation of long sequences of random numbers. He did this by "chunking" the numbers into units that had meaning for him, as he was an avid runner and related them to his running times (one such description appears in Foer 2011). In these pro-nurture books, however, contradictory evidence can often be found – usually in details that the author is not explicitly drawing attention to and curiously does not engage with – that indicates that even with dedicated practise not all individuals will become exceptional performers.

A Japanese forerunner to this is Shinichi Suzuki's (1969) treatise on "Ability Development" which gave rise to the unique Suzuki method of teaching musical instruments, predominantly the violin, to very young children (beginning around the age of three). Suzuki spent his whole career asserting that ability is not inborn (1969; 1983) – a message continuing to be propagated world-wide by the International Suzuki Association – and that any child can develop musical proficiency. However, in Suzuki's message too there is unpublicised "small print". In Book 1 of the teaching manuals that his method relies on, there is this caveat: "The same method may yield different outcomes in different children" (Suzuki 2007:4).

Individual difference

One thing that all the above writers and researchers agree on is that there is difference amongst individuals, as it is patently obvious that not everyone is a Mozart. But they are disagreeing about whether every one of us could be like Mozart if given the same nurture he had. The idea that we all can achieve "greatness" (e.g. Shenk 2010) suggests that we all have constitutionally equal capability that only becomes differentiated through differentiated training – the "blank slate" idea that Pinker (2002) has so cogently critiqued. Whilst this idea is regularly put forward in relation to high ability, marked low ability is, interestingly, typically accepted as a categorisable individual difference rather than construing it as merely a deficit in training or practise. A clear manifestation of this is the persistence of "intellectual disability" as a listed disorder in the regularly revised *Diagnostic and Statistical Manual* of the American Psychiatric Association (2013:33). A diagnosis of intellectual disability is confirmed by IQ testing that yields a score of 70 or lower (American Psychiatric Association 2013:33). Such a diagnosis is therefore predicated upon the idea that intellectual ability is variable, that IQ testing is an appropriate and effective measure of this, and that a certain level of this is considered normal such that impairment in it is listed as a disorder. This status quo is, however, disregarded by the "nurture" authors' thesis that anyone can achieve anything with the right amount of the right kind of practise. Ericsson et al. (2007) does mention that it is the "healthy" individual that has no limits, which then begs the question of how "healthy" is defined.

Loden & Rosener (1990) constructed the "Diversity Wheel" as a way of depicting the differences between people "that are particularly important in shaping our identities" (Lou & Deane, n.d.). Since it first appeared decades ago the Diversity Wheel has been updated by Loden (1995) and others (e.g. Gardenswartz & Rowe 1998), but in its various iterations it has retained as primary the six dimensions that Loden and Rosener (1990) in their original model posited as the core dimensions that constitute "the most powerful and sustaining differences, ones that usually have an important impact on us throughout our lives" (Lou & Deane n.d.), shaping our self-image and worldviews. These are: age, ethnicity, gender, ability, race, and sexual orientation. (To this I would add, as another dimension of individual difference, "neurodiversity", which is a term gaining in presence and which I say more about in Chapter 6.) Each iteration of the Diversity Wheel retains "ability" but in slightly different wordings, e.g. "physical abilities and qualities" (Loden 1995), or "mental/physical ability" (Johns Hopkins University & Medicine n.d.). These various sources accept that ability is a fundamental aspect of a person that varies amongst different people and strongly affects their lives and identities (see also Thomas 1990:50).

Social and interpersonal implications

Mendick (2014) claims that Suzuki misled people with his promise of Ability Development so as "to peddle a method of teaching … that netted him a fortune". Mass popularity and commercial success do seem to back the "nurture" message, as shown by the best-seller status of some of the pro-nurture books mentioned above, and the wide praise for and awards garnered by Gould's (1981) anti-nature book, even though it – and Kamin's (1974) – have since been critiqued as erroneous and refuted. The popularity of the "nurture" message shows that it is what people want to hear, that it is received as inspiring, and that the idea of possible achievement being constrained by biologically determined limits is fiercely resisted.

A favouring of nurture beliefs can certainly lead to positive outcomes by motivating individuals to keep stretching themselves to succeed, and much of worth has been achieved by such means. However, it can also be burdensome and have negative impact. For example, Shenk (2010) explicitly states that it is the parent's responsibility to cultivate "greatness" in their child: holding such a belief will put tremendous pressure on parents, and in turn on children. If parents believe that their child should be able to achieve "greatness" so long as he or she works hard enough, their expectation of that child will be very different than if they hold a belief that inborn abilities determine different limits for different individuals. Although not holding limiting conceptions of what a person might be capable of is usually held up as a good thing (e.g. Stobart 2014), it does have a dark side. A controversial documentation of a parent who relentlessly pushed her children to achieve (Chua 2011) introduced into popular language the term "Tiger Mother" for this phenomenon. (Another similar colloquial term is "stage parent".) Relationships caught up in such a prioritising of driving attainment can become strained and even irreparably damaged, even if great accomplishments have thereby been achieved. One such example in the media is violin celebrity Vanessa-Mae's estrangement from her mother since having sacked her as her manager. And if "greatness" is not achieved a sense of failure can haunt both children and parents, with the attendant destructiveness of disappointment, anger, guilt, shame, and low self-esteem.

Factors in combination

It appears that the anti-nature movement has passed its peak. For example, the debate between Gagné and Ericsson mentioned above (in Kaufman 2013) is formatted so as to give Ericsson with his "nurture" position the advantage of having the last word. A year later he no longer enjoys this editorial advantage: in a special issue (volume 45) of the journal *Intelligence*, eight papers by "experts on expertise" (Detterman 2014) are presented that oppose the arguments and methods of Ericsson. These are followed by a rebuttal by Ericsson (2014), then a response to his rebuttal by the authors of each of the eight papers. Four years after that, two alternative extensive volumes on expertise appeared simultaneously, one by Hambrick et al. (2018), and the other (a second edition) by Ericsson et al. (2018). The first of these two books includes a section on genetic contributions to expertise (nature), whereas the second has no such section and focuses on psychological and sociological perspectives and physiological changes produced by long-term practise (nurture). Each book contains a long list of contributors that – bar two names – is exclusive of the other. So although this reflects the ongoing debate with different adherents to different perspectives, it also highlights how many different factors are involved.

The arguments critiquing the anti-nature position have presented research showing that with the same amount of practise, individuals achieve differently; that practise actually increases the range of individual difference (cited in Gagné 2013); and that deliberate practise alone is not sufficient to achieve expert performance (Hambrick et al. 2014). Exceptional musical performance at very young ages in child prodigies demonstrates that Ericsson's rule of the necessity of 10,000 hours of practise does not apply (Ruthsatz et al. 2014). Neither does it apply in savants who accomplish astounding untrained skill in, for example, drawing (see the case of Stephen Wiltshire, searchable online). Simonton (2009), writing about genius, shows that time spent practising could be inversely proportionate to accomplishment. For example, he cites a study on 120 classical composers which shows that those who took less than the average time in expertise acquisition became more eminent, more prolific, and had longer productive careers. So what is it that accounts for these individual differences?

Ericsson et al. (2007) did concede that sporting achievement could depend on congenital physiological advantages such as height, but insisted that sport was the only domain affected by biological differences. The two most widely studied domains in expertise research are chess and music (Hambrick et al. 2014). It has been shown that chess performance is contributed to independently by practise and by IQ (De Bruin et al. 2014), that expert chess players display significantly higher intelligence than controls, and that their playing strength is related to their intelligence level (Hambrick et al. 2014). In music, child prodigies' abilities have been shown to be highly dependent on higher IQ, exceptional working memory, and elevated attention to detail (Ruthsatz et al. 2014).

Just as practise alone cannot produce exceptional performance, neither can intelligence on its own. No person will achieve outstandingly without the inspiration or "ignition" (Coyle 2010:97) that provokes committing to a particular task, the motivation to sustain that commitment, and the environmental support to continue engaging with that task and continue improving performance. Environmental support includes resources, opportunity, guidance/tuition, and feedback (input from others that identifies which elements can be improved and how so as to optimise performance – Coyle 2010). To these factors Gladwell (2008) added the role of luck, demonstrating how being born at the right time of year in the right historical era and in the right geographical location can give a person advantages in achieving success. (One example he gives is of how such circumstances contributed to Bill Gates's multi-billion dollar success in the computer industry.) So although there is by now a weight of research evidencing intelligence as an important factor in individual difference in performance, from which it could appear that high-IQ individuals are predisposed towards achievement, high intelligence does not necessarily lead to high achievement because of how many other factors are involved. This still leaves the question of whether difference in IQ level itself is innate or not. To address this we move now from research on expertise to research on intelligence.

The trajectory of intelligence research: where it has been and where it might go

Figure 2.1 outlines what I see as the essential questions driving research on intelligence. I will explain the schema and use it as a reference point for summarising the trajectory of such research.

Starting at the top centre of the schema, it can be said of any research field that it has to begin with (1) defining what it is examining. Chapter 1 looked at the defining of intelligence to date. Related to this we traced the history of how (2) a way of measuring intelligence was developed, which for decades has centred on IQ tests. It was also mentioned that new ways of measuring intelligence are being researched that could potentially use brain imaging, DNA testing, or chronometrics instead of IQ tests.

Once intelligence is measured as existing in higher or lower quantities, I see a central question as being (A) "Is it better to have higher intelligence?" The answer "No" could lead to a loss of interest in this as an area for further investigation. However, as already presented, the answer "Yes" has been pointed to by research that has linked higher intelligence with many lifelong positive outcomes. If it is considered therefore that it is indeed better to have higher intelligence, the next logical question

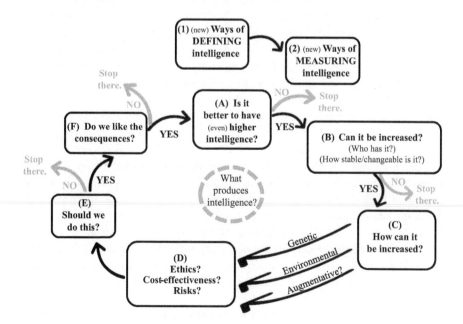

FIGURE 2.1 Intelligence Research schema

is, (B) "Can it be increased?" And this is what I would say is the single most cardinal question that has concertedly driven intelligence research for well over a hundred years, certainly ever since Galton's work on this started in the late 19th century. If there is an interest in increasing intelligence and some people have higher intelligence than others, a related question becomes: "Who has it?" The study of group differences in intelligence is the most contentious area of all in intelligence research. Related to the question of whether intelligence can be increased, is the question of how stable or changeable it is as a trait.

If the answer to "Can intelligence be increased?" is "No", then the research endeavour would end there. To date there has been no conceding that such a conclusion has been reached. Whilst there remains engagement with a belief that "Yes", it is worthwhile to keep trying to increase intelligence, then the next question is, (C) "How can it be increased?" Efforts so far have centred on two main lines of activity, directly reflecting the nature versus nurture debate: genetic versus environmental attempts to increase intelligence. To this I am adding "augmentative" attempts to increase intelligence as a potential new line of activity, which will be explained below. Central to all of this enterprise is the question: "What produces intelligence?"

Any attempted route to increase intelligence brings up questions concerning (D) the related ethics, cost-effectiveness, and risks that are involved. And these questions inevitably lead us to grapple with a deeper question: (E) "Should we do this?" An answer of "No" terminates the related activity. An answer of "Yes" leads us, in trialling further interventions, to the question: (F) "Do we like the consequences?" An answer of "No" would again spell the end of such attempts. An answer of "Yes", however, could lead us again to (A), with the question of whether it is considered to be better to have even higher levels of intelligence. This process could take us clockwise around the research circle again with its sequential questions and possible end points.

In parallel with this activity, it might be that (1) and (2) are also revisited, with new ways of defining intelligence being developed and associated work on potential new ways of measuring this. For example, we have seen already (Chapter 1) how definitions of intelligence as a collection of core cognitive capabilities broadened out over time into definitions of intelligence as including capabilities not confined to the cognitive (Gardner), or as comprising individuals' success at achieving their goals within their sociocultural context (Sternberg). With the latter example, Sternberg developed new methods for measuring what he has defined as successful intelligence, and he has worked (Sternberg 2006) to have the USA's practice of selecting university candidates broadened from solely using SAT tests that measure cognitive abilities to incorporating his tests of candidates' propensities for succeeding through their university education and beyond by additional indices such as practical and creative skills. I wonder about a kind of brave new world in which human intelligence might come to be augmented with brain implantations of computer chips, and such a cyborg product might call for a new definition of intelligence that incorporates the potential new capabilities that the human–machine integration might unleash. What comes to mind is the collaborative mental networking capabilities that distinguish the way the cyborg species "the Borg" operates in the wonderfully imaginative science fiction television series *Star Trek*. With progress of such a kind, new measures of intelligence might also be developed: perhaps ways of measuring the strengths of different implantation types and the processing power produced by different combinations of human–machine integration. It is interesting to speculate about whether the trajectory of intelligence research might possibly lead in such a direction in the future. However, returning to the present, what do we know so far about how intelligence comes about?

What produces intelligence?

Research into the physiological basis of intelligence has been rapidly advanced by brain imaging technologies introduced since the 1980s – such as PET scans (Positron Emission Tomography), structural Magnetic Resonance Imaging (MRI), and Functional MRI (fMRI) – that have made it possible to directly examine the living human brain. Biological correlates for intelligence have been confirmed in both the structure and functioning of the brain (Geake 2009; Haier 2017). Brain size (cranial capacity), volume of grey matter, and density of white matter have all been shown to increase with increasing intelligence (several studies cited in Haier 2017). Giftedness has been correlated with neural efficiency, with studies evidencing that in higher IQ less cortical activity is necessary to learn a new task (Grabner et al. 2003), with more efficient use of brain resources such as glucose metabolism (i.e. consuming less energy) (Haier et al. 1988; Vitouch et al. 1997; Jausovec 2000; Neubauer et al. 2002). The Parieto-Frontal Integration Theory (PFIT) emphasises that as well as having identified the parietal and frontal areas as being the specific brain areas most strongly involved in intelligence, it is the networks that link these and the efficiency of the interactions between them that is key (Haier 2017). Another finding, using neuroimaging together with advanced genetic analysis in very large samples, has been that many of the brain characteristics associated with intelligence are under genetic control (Haier 2017).

Prior to the availability of these research techniques the predominant method of researching genetic contributions to intelligence was the use of twin studies, where similarity in intelligence between identical or monozygotic (MZ) twins, who share all their DNA, was compared with that of fraternal or dizygotic (DZ) twins, who only share half of their DNA (Haier 2017). Findings – with different exact figures in different studies depending particularly on the twins' age at testing – have been that MZ twins have a much higher correlation in IQ (over 0.80) than DZ twins do (around 0.60) (Haier 2017), or than other siblings or parent–child pairs do (below 0.50) (Hunt 2011). Similar results have also been replicated by using a newer methodology called Genome-wide Complex Trait Analysis (GCTA) which directly compares the DNA between any individuals, thereby overcoming criticisms that have been made of the design of twin studies

(Ritchie 2015). The conclusion is that in adulthood intelligence has over 80% heritability (heritability being the percentage of variation in a trait, in a given population, that is accounted for by genetics) (Hunt 2011; Haier 2017). This means that general intelligence has one of the highest heritabilities of any human characteristic (Simonton 2009).

It is quantitative genetics that measures how much genes make a difference to a particular trait, and molecular genetics that tries to identify which genes are responsible for the differences. Whilst specific genes have been identified for certain conditions – such as phenylketonuria (PKU) – that are associated with mental disability, it has been harder to find specific genes for general intelligence (Mackintosh 2011). Some genes showing direct correlation with intelligence have begun to be discovered (see Haier 2017), but what has been ascertained is that intelligence is polygenic, meaning that many genes are involved, each having a small effect (Haier 2017). This makes sense given the number of different elements and processes that comprise intelligence. Researching this is particularly complicated as it depends on consortia of international research groups collaborating so as to gather large enough samples for any trends to become visible (Haier 2017). I find it remarkable that there is such a desire to try to acquire this kind of causal knowledge that such extensive efforts are being invested in.

A further complexity in genetics is that it is not about the mere presence or absence of particular genes, but about how genes express themselves – whether they are switched on or off – which can change over a lifespan and is affected by external influences: this is the domain of epigenetics. Understanding how this works in intelligence will require much more research (Haier 2017), but it is here where outcomes are influenced by how environmental factors interact with genes. However high the genetic heritability of intelligence is, it is never 100%. A person's genetic composition determines their "reaction range" (Hunt 2011:24), meaning the range of intelligence levels that is possible for that person, and then it is the quality of the environment that will determine where within that range the person's functioning will be.

Anything in the environment – prenatal and postnatal – that damages the structure of the brain or interferes with brain processing can reduce intelligence. This includes injury, disease, environmental toxins, and substance use. Examples of relevant research findings that are well-established and unequivocal, are that maternal alcohol consumption during pregnancy significantly negatively impacts foetal intellectual development; that higher birth-weight is correlated with higher intelligence; and that prolonged malnutrition lowers IQ scores, as does exposure to lead in the atmosphere (see Hunt 2011).

Looking beyond these purely physical factors, research on environmental effects on intelligence has also used twin studies. Tests have been carried out on the similarity in IQ between MZ twins raised together in the same environment versus those who have been separated at birth and raised in different environments. The results of such tests have been compared with similarity in IQ between DZ twins – and biologically unrelated individuals – raised together or apart. A striking finding has been that the heritability of intelligence increases with increasing age (Hunt 2011; Ritchie 2015; Haier 2017). What this means is that shared environments (family and home influences) and non-shared environments (influences outside of the family and home such as teachers, friends, and activities experienced) have some effect on IQ during childhood but the effects of shared environments disappear entirely by the age of 16 and the effects of non-shared environments wane so that from age 18 onwards they have an impact of less than 20% (Haier 2017). The explanation of this is that children cannot choose the environment they are brought up in, but when they are adults and do choose their environment, they choose according to their (genetically determined) level of intelligence (Haier 2017). Individuals with higher IQ choose to be in more complex and intellectually stimulating environments. The conclusion from this is that shared and non-shared environments have little lasting effect on levels of intelligence.

Related to this, is that correlations found between higher IQ and higher socioeconomic status (SES) are often assumed to be a "nurture" effect – i.e. it is assumed that higher SES produces increased intelligence. However, a weight of research evidence supports this correlation being more of a "nature" effect: as mentioned in Chapter 1, people with higher intelligence generally stay in education for longer plus learn more (Hunt 2011), leading to higher educational attainment, which is often a prerequisite for the securing of more complex and intellectually demanding jobs, which generally produce higher income, leading to higher SES. Children in higher SES homes who also have higher IQ are apparently manifesting the benefits of their genetic heritage of their parents' intelligence to a greater extent than they are manifesting the benefits conferred by the more privileged lifestyles their parents are providing for them (Hunt 2011; Ritchie 2015; Haier 2017:55–56 & 192–196). A caution in such research, however, is that there is not one uniform method for defining and measuring SES. So whilst different studies refer to SES as though it is known what this is, what exact factors have been measured and how these have been interpreted varies (Hunt 2011).

Who has it?

If it is perceived that it is better to have higher rather than lower intelligence, and humans are placed in groups according to categories named as race and ethnicity, and then some of those groups are said to have higher or lower intelligence than others, it easily leads – and notoriously has led – to such groups becoming correspondingly stereotyped and treated with discrimination as though some are better or worse (rather than only having higher or lower intelligence) than others. Because of this, I have not so far been able to be convinced that there is any good reason to seek information about how mean levels of intelligence might compare across different geographical regions or group divisions, especially given the fact that intelligence cannot currently be measured on a ratio scale in the way that an individual difference like height can be. Also, once any grouping is made it can be fiendishly problematic to determine which individuals do or do not have membership of that group: the Apartheid Museum in South Africa documents the extensive problems that country encountered when trying to classify individuals into the racial groups its regime had constructed in order to enforce its race-based legislation.

If information on so-called group differences is sought, what to do with it once acquired becomes an issue. Using such information to set policies or practices in any domain in any way that is based solely on perceived membership of constructed groups can never be just. And very often it is not actually factual information that drives the way that different groups or perceived members of different groups are treated, but power dynamics or social agendas. An extreme example of this is that when Hitler set out to build a superior race, he held up higher intelligence as part of human excellence. However, he also set out to destroy Jews, when factual information evidenced by research is that Jews have particularly high intelligence and are overrepresented in many areas of achievement including in the winning of Nobel Prizes (Lynn & Longley 2006). Hitler's focus on propagating white-skinned, blue-eyed, blond-haired Aryans reveals his primary agenda as having been about advancing power for his own ethnicity. And it could be construed, in his attempt to destroy a group who have been found to have markedly high intelligence, that it was the threat they posed to the prospects of dominance for his own group that he was actually trying to eliminate. The way that these kinds of atrocity, discrimination, and problems with accurate classification plague the naming of group differences is why I would prefer to prevent data about race or ethnicity ever being collected in matters to do with intelligence – and indeed in all other matters I can think of also, such as in educational and employment contexts. I am open to being corrected on this, but as far as I can currently see it is only in purely medical contexts that the collecting of such data is warranted, as it can be helpful to know about which specific genetic and health risks and vulnerabilities have been scientifically linked with different ethnicities.

How stable or changeable is intelligence?

Individual IQ has been shown to remain mostly stable over time (Schneider et al. 2014). There is, however, deterioration in older age (Deary et al. 2009; Hunt 2011), with the effects on Gf being more marked than on Gc. (And it has been evidenced that people who have one type of the $APOE$ gene have lower intelligence in later life as well as faster mental decline with age – cited in Ritchie 2015.) Change in ability (rather than IQ specifically) can come about in other ways: it can be enhanced through long-term deliberate practise (Ericsson et al. 1993; 2018), or – as documented in the case of New York orthopaedic surgeon Tony Cicoria – suddenly expand remarkably through a rare accident. Cicoria, after having survived being struck by lightning, found himself having a completely new compulsion and ability to play the piano and compose music, without former training, and dropped his medical career to pursue instead a career as a classical musician (Sacks 2007). An equally sudden loss in intelligence can be incurred through the sustaining of traumatic brain injury (Arciniegas et al. 2002).

The much-mentioned Flynn Effect refers to James Flynn's studies which showed that average IQ scores within the populations of many Western industrialised nations had steadily increased during the 20th century (Flynn 1984; 1987). This finding has largely been attributable to a rise in the lowest IQ range which has pushed up the mean figure (Hunt 2011). One likely factor producing this effect is improved foetal and infant nutrition and health (Lynn 1998): this phenotypic improvement (improving the environmental interaction with genetic potential) clearly does not affect the highest IQ range where genotype or genetic potential is already being optimally expressed. In the 21st century, however, the reverse effect has been documented: drops in IQ scores have been recorded in many nations including Australia, Denmark, Norway, the United Kingdom (studies cited in Kanazawa 2012:189), and in German-speaking countries (Pietschnig & Gittler 2015). It has been hypothesised that this observed decrease – termed the Negative Flynn Effect – has resulted from a ceiling having been reached in the improvements to intelligence that can be produced by better nutrition (Kanazawa 2012) and other phenotypic effects (Dutton et al. 2016). What this means is that what is now becoming exposed is genotypic deterioration through the dysgenic effect of higher-IQ men and women preferring to have no children (Kanazawa 2012) and higher intelligence being correlated with lower rates of reproduction (Kanazawa 2012; Meisenberg 2010).

Attempts to increase intelligence: genetic, environmental, augmentative?

Trying to increase intelligence through genetic methods is what eugenics was about, as described in Chapter 1. Applying such practices to whole populations at a policy level is no longer tolerated as ethical, and rightly so. However, at an individual level – outside of intelligence being a factor that operates naturally, even if not consciously, in mate selection (Mascie-Taylor & Vandenberg 1988) – contemporary reproductive technologies do provide opportunities for making more deliberate choices about this. For example, standard antenatal practices in many countries now allow for the likelihood of conditions such as Down syndrome to be tested for, and, if test results are positive, for termination to be offered. When donor sperm or eggs are used in conception, IQ is one of the factors that can be taken into account in selecting which donor to use. Pre-implantation genetic diagnosis is already used during in vitro fertilisation (IVF) procedures to screen embryos for monogenic disorders like Huntington's disease (Bostrom 2014). Genetic engineering on a larger scale could be possible with the new CRISPR/Cas9 technique of using bacteria to edit the genome of living cells by making changes to targeted genes (cited in Haier 2017:164). But for this to work, the specific genes needing to be targeted in order to affect intelligence with this method would first have to be confirmed and that, as discussed, is a colossal challenge. However, the more that any such methods are used not to prevent health problems but to design preferred forms of life, the more we are led back to forms of eugenics and the more strongly the question arises of the ethics of making use of such methods.

Environmental attempts to increase intelligence have focused on improving the physical factors mentioned above, such as tackling disease and environmental pollutants and improving health and nutrition during pregnancy and childhood. For example, campaigns to encourage new mothers to breastfeed, citing increased intelligence in infants who are breastfed, have been widespread in the UK, although the research evidence for whether breastfeeding actually increases intelligence is mixed (e.g. Isaacs et al. 2010 and Horta et al. 2015 say it does, whereas Girard et al. 2017 say it does not). A nutritional factor with completely unmixed, strong research evidence is that severe iodine deficiency can lead to a loss of nearly a full standard deviation in IQ points (see Bostrom 2014:44). Iodine deficiency affects up to two billion individuals in impoverished inland areas of the world, and can be prevented simply and inexpensively through fortification of table salt (Bostrom 2014:44). Taking other dietary supplements – like omega-3 – has been popularly encouraged but I have not been able to find research that conclusively demonstrates an impact on IQ. Neither do cognitive enhancement drugs impact IQ: these have limited evidence for efficacy in improving attention, learning, and memory, but their use also comes with medical risks and numerous ethical issues (see Haier 2017:157). Haier (2017) describes the researching of new techniques of non-invasive brain stimulation using magnetic fields, electric currents, and cold lasers to improve cognitive performance. Some successes have been reported with these, but also, alarmingly, the use of some such methods actually returned results of reduced IQ test performance (Haier 2017), which highlights the risks involved. In order to build conclusive results there will need to be many more high-quality and independently replicated studies, including studies of the long-term effects of use of any such methods.

Non-physiological environmental interventions to increase intelligence have included attempts to enrich childhood stimuli with targeted toys, books, computer games, and even particular trends such as playing Mozart to young babies, or attempts to increase adult intelligence by engaging in memory training. None of these have been evidenced to alter IQ (related studies are comprehensively reviewed in Haier 2017). The largest and most intensive environmental initiatives to increase intelligence have been early educational programmes such as Head Start in the US (Hunt 2011). These have been shown to produce an increase of only a few IQ points, with the increase disappearing after the intervention ended – termed the "fade-out effect" (Hunt 2011; Protzko 2015). Although increase in IQ was not substantial nor sustained, other positive effects were documented such as fewer social and behavioural problems and higher rates of entry to college than in the control group (Hunt 2011). In terms of actual level of IQ, however, it has become evident that it is on the whole easier for environmental influences to harm rather than to enhance intelligence. The question of cost-effectiveness arises in relation to environmental interventions to increase intelligence given that the expense and intense effort involved have so far produced minimal results.

If neither genetic, nor environmental, attempts to increase intelligence have yielded incontrovertible as well as ethical long-term successes, are there any other possibilities? The idea was mentioned above of possible augmentative attempts to increase intelligence with, for example, cyborg-type implants. With any such idea the questions arise again of the ethics, cost-effectiveness, and risks involved. Nick Bostrom, professor at the University of Oxford and a director of both the Future of Humanity Institute and the Strategic Artificial Intelligence Research Centre, sees the development of a brain–computer interface as very unlikely because of the neurosurgical complications involved such as infection, electrode displacement, haemorrhage, and cognitive decline (Bostrom 2014). Apart from the physiological risks involved, there are risks involved in changing humanity as we currently know it. What consequences this might lead to, and whether or not we would like the consequences, is unknown.

An analogy encapsulating the main issues

The main issues covered in this chapter can be encapsulated by comparing human intelligence with computers. The physical components of a computer's hardware – its CPU (Central Processing Unit) plus storage space or RAM (Random Access Memory) – are like the physical structure of the brain, and the hardware's functionability is analogous to fluid intelligence (Gf). The computer's hardware composition – or the person's (genetically influenced) brain composition – provides the basic physical foundation from which the functioning potential or "reaction range" arises.

Computer software constitutes the programs that are loaded into the computer, as additions to its hardware foundation. This is like crystallised intelligence (Gc) – the knowledge and skills that a person acquires. The quality of the software – just like the quality of a person's education – affects what performance is possible. A fast CPU with ample RAM but only rudimentary software will not be able to perform very complex tasks. Similarly, more limited hardware will not perform very efficiently or have the capacity to make full use of sophisticated software. In the same way, a person's brain biology circumscribes the level of intellectual complexity that he or she is capable of: limited neurological functioning will not support full engagement with sophisticated educational input, and powerful neurological capability will not achieve very much if all it has access to is rudimentary knowledge and skill.

How a computer's user interacts with the computer determines how much of what the hardware is capable of will be demanded of it, what software will be added to it, and how the combined hardware and software will be given the opportunity to perform interesting or complex tasks and be further updated and adapted or not. The computer user is analogous to the environment in which a person finds him- or herself: a person's environment will to differing degrees interact with what he or she is capable of. A more advanced computer user can draw greater functionality out of a mediocre computer than a less advanced user can draw out of a sophisticated computer. In the same way, a person with lower IQ who is fully engaged by a rich environment will achieve more than will a person with higher IQ who is neglected within an impoverished environment. If, however, both of those persons are fully supported to achieve their best in a rich and engaging environment then the person with higher IQ will outperform the other. An important difference, though, is that whilst common passive computers cannot choose their user, people do have the possibility of choosing different environments for themselves.

A person's outwardly noticeable appearance – such as skin and eye colour, hair, body shape and size, grooming and dress – is analogous to the casing and outward appearance of a computer, and a person's ethnicity and nationality is analogous to a computer's branding. People have associations to a computer's appearance and brand, and will find an Apple, say, desirable or undesirable to the extent that they have an affinity with or aversion to what is associated with that brand and its reputation. In the same way, people have associations to individuals' outward appearances and ethnicities and nationalities and they exhibit preferences and develop stereotypes about these. Someone might want an Apple rather than a PC, even if the PC is less expensive and superior in its functionality, because they assume the Apple is better based on what it looks like or its brand status. In addition, software brands are similar to educational brands. Certain combinations of outward appearance, ethnicity or nationality, and educational brand (e.g. a Harvard degree) will be particularly desirable to some: this is like "old boys" networks, where alumni of specific institutions are immediately recognised and trusted as reliable "products", and might be given preference – in recruitment decisions for example – over more unfamiliar "products" that might be as good or even better but do not (yet) have the benefit of having a known and trusted reputation, or being associated with favourable status. Similarly, the presumed-to-be preferential product might disappoint and the confidence in it turn out to be misplaced.

Summary

This chapter has engaged with the nature versus nurture debate on what produces outstanding performance, looking at research on expertise and on intelligence. The popularity of the "nurture" message has been considered and its implications in, for example, the Tiger Mother phenomenon. Classifications of individual difference have been discussed with reference to the Diversity Wheel, to which it has been suggested an addition should be made of "neurodiversity" as another dimension of individual difference. An original schema has been presented that shows the essential questions driving intelligence research to date and how this might develop in the future, together with the related issues of the ethics, cost-effectiveness, and risks involved. Areas summarised include the latest neurological and genetic findings on intelligence, the effects of SES, and the stability/changeability of intelligence over time, including the Flynn Effect and Negative Flynn Effect. Attempts to increase intelligence have been reviewed. The chapter has ended with a computer analogy of how intelligence, performance, appearances, and social assumptions relate to each other.

The point of documenting here and perhaps even emphasising the extent to which intelligence is a neurobiological trait with major genetic influence, is to remind us of this dimension which has been broadly neglected because of the abhorrent history associated with it and its resultant unpopularity and political sensitivity. For example, Warne et al.'s (2018) analysis of intelligence-related content in 29 psychology textbooks found that these contained an uncritically presented bias towards environmental explanations of individual differences in intelligence. Taking the neurobiological dimension into account is necessary in order to avoid the injustice of treating individuals who have particularly low or extremely high IQ as though their manifest ability is only a social construction and correspondingly expect that with enough personal effort or appropriate social policy the differences can be eliminated.

Whatever we call it, think or feel about it, or attribute it to, it is a reality that there are variable levels of attainment noticeable amongst age peers in any given environment. From my perspective it does not actually matter what has caused a person to stand out for high performance, because my main interest is in how the fact of someone standing out in this way is noticed and reacted to and affects people. The construct of high ability is always dependent on a social event – an event in which the performance of someone is judged by an observer as being in some way exceptional relative to that with which that observer is familiar. However, the beliefs people hold about what causes the observed differences, and how this should be dealt with, will affect their intrapersonal and interpersonal feelings and behaviours, and it is these that we will study in the next chapters.

References

American Psychiatric Association. (2013). *Diagnostic and Statistical Manual of Mental Disorders: DSM-5*. (5th ed.). Washington, DC: American Psychiatric Publishing.

Arciniegas, D. B., Held, K. & Wagner, P. (2002). Cognitive impairment following traumatic brain injury. *Current Treatment Options in Neurology*, 4(1), pp. 43–57.

Bostrom, N. (2014). *Superintelligence*. Oxford: Oxford University Press.

Chua, A. (2011). *Battle Hymn of the Tiger Mother*. London: Bloomsbury.

Colvin, G. (2008). *Talent Is Overrated – What Really Separates World-Class Performers from Everybody Else*. London: Nicholas Brealey Publishing.

Coyle, D. (2010). *The Talent Code – Greatness Isn't Born. It's Grown*. London: Arrow Books.

Deary, I. J., Corley, J., Gow, A. J., Harris, S. E., Houlihan, L. M., Marioni, R. E., Penke, L., Rafnsson, S. B. & Starr, J. M. (2009). Age-associated cognitive decline. *British Medical Bulletin*, 92(1), pp. 135–152.

De Bruin, A. B. H., Kok, E. M., Leppink, J. & Camp, G. (2014). Practice, intelligence, and enjoyment in novice chess players: a prospective study at the earliest stage of a chess career. *Intelligence*, 45, pp. 18–25.

Detterman, D. K. (2014). Introduction to the intelligence special issue on the development of expertise: is ability necessary? *Intelligence*, 45, pp. 1–5.

Dutton, E., van der Linden, D. & Lynn, R. (2016). The negative Flynn Effect: a systematic literature review. *Intelligence*, 59, pp. 163–169.

Ericsson, A. K. (2014). Why expert performance is special and cannot be extrapolated from studies of performance in the general population: a response to criticisms. *Intelligence*, 45, pp. 81–103.

Ericsson, K. A., Hoffman, R. R., Kozbelt, A. & Williams, A. M. (Eds.). (2018). *The Cambridge Handbook of Expertise and Expert Performance*. (2nd ed.). Cambridge: Cambridge University Press.

Ericsson, K. A., Krampe, R. T. & Tesch-Romer, C. (1993). The role of deliberate practice in the acquisition of expert performance. *Psychological Review*, 100, pp. 364–403.

Ericsson, K. A., Roring, R. W. & Nandagopal, K. (2007). Giftedness and evidence for reproducibly superior performance: an account based on the expert-performance framework. *High Ability Studies*, 18, pp. 3–56.

Flynn, J. R. (1984). The mean IQ of Americans: massive gains 1932 to 1978. *Psychological Bulletin*, 95, pp. 29–51.

Flynn, J. R. (1987). Massive IQ gains in 14 nations: what IQ tests really measure. *Psychological Bulletin*, 101, pp. 171–191.

Foer, J. (2011). *Moonwalking with Einstein: The Art and Science of Remembering Everything*. London: Penguin.

Gagné, F. (2013). Yes, giftedness (aka "innate" talent) does exist! In: S. B. Kaufman (Ed.). *The Complexity of Greatness*. Oxford: Oxford University Press. pp. 191–221.

Galton, F. (1869). *Hereditary Genius: An Inquiry into Its Causes and Consequences*. London: Macmillan.

Galton, F. (1874). *English Men of Science: Their Nature and Nurture*. London: Macmillan.

Gardenswartz, L. & Rowe, A. (1998). *Managing Diversity: A Complete Desk Reference and Planning Guide*. New York: McGraw-Hill.

Geake, J. G. (2009). Neuropsychological characteristics of academic and creative giftedness. In: L. V. Shavinina (Ed.). *International Handbook on Giftedness*. Quebec: Springer. pp. 261–273.

Girard, L.-C., Doyle, O. & Tremblay, R. E. (2017). Breastfeeding, cognitive and noncognitive development in early childhood: a population study. *Pediatrics*, 139(4). Published online: 10.1542/peds.2016-1848.

Gladwell, M. (2008). *Outliers: The Story of Success*. London: Allen Lane.

Gould, S. J. (1981). *The Mismeasure of Man*. New York: W. W. Norton & Company.

Grabner, R. H., Stern, E. & Neubauer, A. C. (2003). When intelligence loses its impact: neural efficiency during reasoning in a familiar area. *International Journal of Psychophysiology*, 49, pp. 89–98.

Haier, R. J. (2017). *The Neuroscience of Intelligence*. Cambridge: Cambridge University Press.

Haier, R. J., Siegel, B. V., Nuechterlein, K. H., Hazlett, E., Wu, J. C., Paek, J., Browning, H. L. & Buchsbaum, M. S. (1988). Cortical glucose metabolic rate correlates of abstract reasoning and attention studied with positron emission tomography. *Intelligence*, 12, pp. 199–217.

Hambrick, D. Z., Campitelli, G. & Macnamara, B. N. (2018). *The Science of Expertise*. New York: Routledge.

Hambrick, D. Z., Oswald, F. L., Altmann, E. M., Meinz, E. J., Gobet, F. & Campitelli, G. (2014). Deliberate practice: is that all it takes to become an expert? *Intelligence*, 45, pp. 34–45.

Herrnstein, R. J. & Murray, C. (1994). *The Bell Curve: Intelligence and Class Structure in American Life*. New York: Free Press Paperbacks.

Horta, B. L., de Mola, C. L. & Victora, C. G. (2015). Breastfeeding and intelligence: a systematic review and meta-analysis. *Acta Paediatrica*, 104(S467). Published online: 10.1111/apa.13139.

Howe, M. J. A., Davidson, J. W. & Sloboda, J. A. (1998). Innate talents: reality or myth? *Behavioural and Brain Sciences*, 21, pp. 399–442.

Hunt, E. (2011). *Human Intelligence*. New York: Cambridge University Press.

Isaacs, E. B., Fischl, B. R., Quinn, B. T., Chong, W. K., Gadian, D. G. & Lucas, A. (2010). Impact of breast milk on intelligence quotient, brain size and white matter development. *Pediatric Research*, 67, pp. 357–362.

Jausovec, N. (2000). Differences in cognitive processes between gifted, intelligent, creative, and average individuals while solving complex problems: an EEG study. *Intelligence*, 28, pp. 213–237.

Johns Hopkins University & Medicine. (n.d.). *Diversity Wheel*. [online] Available at: http://web.jhu.edu/dlc/resources/diversity_wheel/ [Accessed 28 December 2016].

Kamin, L. (1974). *The Science and Politics of IQ*. New York: Routledge.

Kanazawa, S. (2012). *The Intelligence Paradox*. Hoboken, NJ: John Wiley & Sons.

Kaufman, S. B. (Ed.) (2013). *The Complexity of Greatness – Beyond Talent or Practice*. Oxford: Oxford University Press.

Lawrence, C. (2003). *The Roman Mysteries: The Enemies of Jupiter*. London: Orion.

Loden, M. (1995). *Implementing Diversity*. New York: McGraw-Hill.

Loden, M. & Rosener, J. (1990). *Workforce America! Managing Employee Diversity as a Vital Resource*. New York: McGraw-Hill.

Lou, K. & Deane, B. (n.d.). *Signs of Change: Global Diversity Puts New Spin on Loden's Diversity Wheel*. [online] Available at: www.loden.com/Web_Stuff/Articles_-_Videos_Survey/Entries/2010/9/3_Global_Diversity_Puts_New_Spin_on_Lodens_Diversity_Wheel.html. [Accessed 28 December 2016].

Lynn, R. (1998). In support of the nutrition theory. In: U. Neisser (Ed.). *The Rising Curve: Long-Term Gains in IQ and Related Measures*. Washington, DC: American Psychological Association, pp. 207–215.

Lynn, R. & Longley, D. (2006). On the high intelligence and cognitive achievements of Jews in Britain. *Intelligence*, 34(6), pp. 541–547.

Mackintosh, N. J. (2011). *IQ and Human Intelligence*. (2nd ed.). Oxford: Oxford University Press.

Mascie-Taylor, C. G. N. & Vandenberg, S. G. (1988). Assortative mating for IQ and personality due to propinquity and personal preference. *Behavior Genetics*, 18(3), pp. 339–345.

Meisenberg, G. (2010). The reproduction of intelligence. *Intelligence*, 38, pp. 220–230.

Mendick, R. (2014). Violin teacher Suzuki is the biggest fraud in music history, says expert. *The Telegraph*. [online] Available at: www.telegraph.co.uk/news/worldnews/asia/japan/11188226/Violin-teacher-Suzuki-is-the-biggest-fraud-in-music-history-says-expert.html. [Accessed 4 January 2017].

Neubauer, A. C., Fink, A. & Schrausser, D. G. (2002). Intelligence and neural efficiency: the influence of task content and sex on brain–IQ relationship. *Intelligence*, 30, pp. 515–536.

Nobel Laureates Facts. (n.d.). [online] Available at: www.nobelprize.org/prizes/facts/nobel-prize-facts. [Accessed 7 April 2019].

Pietschnig, J. & Gittler, G. (2015). A reversal of the Flynn effect for spatial perception in German-speaking countries: evidence from a cross-temporal IRT-based meta-analysis (1977–2014). *Intelligence*, 53, pp. 145–153.

Pinker, S. (2002). *The Blank Slate*. London: Penguin.

Protzko, J. (2015). The environment in raising early intelligence: a meta-analysis of the fadeout effect. *Intelligence*, 53, pp. 202–210.

Ritchie, S. J. (2015). *Intelligence – All That Matters*. London: John Murray Learning.

Ruthsatz, J., Ruthsatz, K. & Ruthsatz Stephens, K. (2014). Putting practice into perspective: child prodigies as evidence of innate talent. *Intelligence*, 45, pp. 60–65.

Sacks, O. (2007). A bolt from the blue. *The New Yorker*. 23 July issue.

Schneider, W., Niklas, F. & Schmiedeler, S. (2014). Intellectual development from early childhood to early adulthood: the impact of early IQ differences on stability and change over time. *Learning and Individual Differences*, 32, pp. 156–162.

Shenk, D. (2010). *The Genius in All of Us – Why Everything You've Been Told About Genetics, Talent and Intelligence Is Wrong*. London: Icon Books.

Simonton, D. K. (2009). *Genius 101*. New York: Springer.

Sternberg, R. J. (2006). The Rainbow Project: enhancing the SAT through assessments of analytical, practical, and creative skills. *Intelligence*, 34(4), pp. 321–350.

Stobart, G. (2014). *The Expert Learner: Challenging the Myth of Ability*. Berkshire, UK: Open University Press.

Suzuki, S. (1969). *Ability Development from Age Zero*. Translated from the Japanese by M. L. Nagata. Reprint 1981. Miami, FL: Summy-Birchard Music.

Suzuki, S. (1983). *Nurtured by Love – The Classic Approach to Talent Education*. (2nd ed.). Translated from the Japanese by W. Suzuki. Miami, FL: Warner Bros. Publications.

Suzuki, S. (2007). *Suzuki Violin School Volume 1 Violin Part*. Los Angeles, CA: Summy-Birchard Inc.

Syed, M. (2010). *Bounce: How Champions are Made*. London: Fourth Estate.

Thomas, R. M. (1990). *Counseling and Life-Span Development*. London: Sage.

Vitouch, O., Bauer, H., Gittler, G., Leodolter, M. & Leodolter, U. (1997). Cortical activity of good and poor spatial test performers during spatial and verbal processing studied with slow potential topography. *International Journal of Psychophysiology*, 27, pp. 183–199.

Warne, R. T., Astle, M. C. & Hill, J. C. (2018). What do undergraduates learn about human intelligence? An analysis of introductory psychology textbooks. *Archives of Scientific Psychology*, 6, pp. 32–50.

3

CORE BIOPSYCHOSOCIAL ISSUES

Needing to be noticed, dreading rejection

> **Reflective Prompt 3:** Imagine that a new person is coming into your personal or professional life, and you hear this person described as being extremely intelligent. What is your immediate reaction? How do you anticipate this person will behave towards you, and you towards him or her? Can you describe any benefit you would expect from this situation? Or any threat? Would your response to this have been different at different times in your life?

This chapter bridges Part I and Part II of the book: it continues Part I's "development" theme by looking at the core issues affecting our psychosocial development through the human biological lifespan, but in outlining these issues also prepares for Part II's "predicaments" theme by providing foundational concepts that situate high-IQ individuals' social interactions within a wider framework of mainstream psychological theory. The chapter looks at extreme intelligence as something extraordinary that co-exists with ordinary general human lifespan development, emphasising the importance of person–environment interaction, the need to be noticed or recognised and find belonging, and the centrality of interpersonal relating. For clarity I have organised these ideas into an overview model titled "High-IQ Context" (Figure 3.1), and the chapter is structured around explaining this model.

The "High-IQ Context" model

In summary, this model depicts a *person* (in this case an extremely high-IQ person) existing within an *environment* with which reciprocal *recognition* and *interaction* are constantly taking place. Learning occurs from such interaction, forming

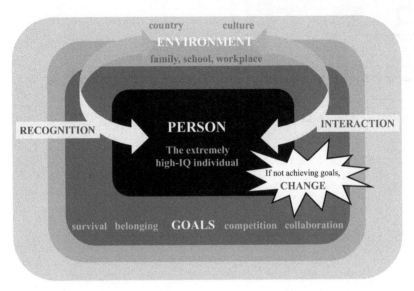

FIGURE 3.1 High-IQ Context model

habits and expectations, and impelling the individual to effect *change* to the self and/or the environment as may become necessary for the achieving of biopsychosocial *goals*. This model (in Figure 3.1) therefore contains constitutive elements (in white lettering – person, environment, goals) plus the related dynamic processes (in black lettering – recognition, interaction, change). Each of these will be discussed in the next sections.

Goals: survival, belonging, competition, collaboration

The first goal of any organism is survival. The human infant is born helpless, vulnerable, and utterly dependent for its survival on being noticed by and having its needs recognised and responded to by an other – principally usually a mother. Such needs include being provided with protection, nutrition, and even, initially, regulation of body temperature (see Winberg 2005). Being rejected, or abandoned, at this stage would almost certainly mean death, as shown by the Ancient Roman practice of "exposure" (see Harris 1994) whereby unwanted babies were left alone outdoors overnight to die. As argued by Object Relations and Attachment theorists and evidenced by the neuroscience of intersubjectivity (e.g. see Schore 2016), infants enter the world genetically programmed to seek security by establishing relationships with caregivers who can recognise, protect, and provide for them.

As the human grows and matures, other goals develop such as those of pairing, generating, and nurturing. These goals are associated with the unfolding of our genetic design, with biologically punctuated milestones such as the production of certain hormones setting in or increasing (for example during puberty) or ceasing (for example during the female menopause). The concomitant physiological and psychosocial processes that are experienced have to be navigated, from childhood growth spurts through to the maturation of adult sexuality and finally the progression through old age and dying.

When the fundamental survival-related goals are met, other goals can arise. This is what Humanistic theorist Abraham Maslow (1943) depicted in his famous model of the Hierarchy of Needs. The need that can be called the most privileged of needs, as it is the one that arises only when all the others in the hierarchy have already been met, is the need for what Maslow called "self-actualisation" (1943). This entails seeking self-fulfilment through realising one's potentials. Psychodynamic theorist Erik Erikson (1950) built a widely cited eight-stage theory of how different psychosocial goals typically play out over the lifespan of the human being whose basic needs of safety and nutrition are being adequately met.

The key elements of Attachment Theory correspond with the above outline of the human lifecourse. Psychologist, psychiatrist, and psychoanalyst John Bowlby (1969; 1973; 1980) theorised the "attachment system" as a genetically programmed regulatory system that governs from birth onwards the human infant's seeking of security through sophisticatedly nuanced interpersonal relating that is designed to maximise the meeting of needs for safety and belonging. Infants quickly adapt to who their available caregivers are, optimising the strategies that they learn are most reliable in eliciting the attention they need. The kind of response from significant others that the infant predominantly experiences establishes what Bowlby (1969) termed an "internal working model", which is like a map that predicts what to expect of people based on previous experience. The internal working model accordingly shapes what patterns of interaction – or "attachment styles" (Ainsworth et al. 1978; Bartholomew & Horowitz 1991) – the infant will predominantly use in relating with others. Once a person's attachment style has developed it remains largely stable throughout life unless disrupted by specific intervention or intense experience (Howe 2011).

When a threat to a person's security is perceived it is said that the attachment system is activated, and this triggers the well-known "fight, flight, or freeze" response (Cannon 1939). A visceral fear persists throughout life – felt and expressed more or less keenly at different developmental stages – of loss of the protective other who is termed "the secure base" (Bowlby 1988), with whom there is an enduring affectional tie or attachment relationship, and to whom a maintaining of proximity is sought. Separation from the secure base arouses protest and distress (Bowlby et al. 1952; Bowlby 1988), which at its original and most extreme form is distress at a perceived threat to survival. The infant's attachment system correlates with the parent's caregiving system, and humans who are in an attachment relationship with each other have been evidenced to form a co-regulating unit where the physiological, psychological, and emotional states of one become synchronised with those of the other and reciprocally affect each other (Stern 1985; Sroufe 1989). These relational experiences sculpt the baby's developing brain, with lifelong implications (Gerhardt 2015). Compelling research evidence on this neuroscience of intersubjectivity has multiplied in recent years (e.g. see Schore 2016). At around puberty the adolescent shifts his or her primary attachment from his or her parents or other adult caregivers to peers. At this stage pair bonds (romantic relationships – see Hazan & Shaver 1987) are sought and established and with the maturation of the adolescent's own caregiving system and biological capacity to reproduce, he or she in turn might procreate and nurture new infants.

From an evolutionary perspective, it is those humans who learned to group together to help each other to secure safety from predators and to secure resources such as food and shelter who were more successful at survival, and this has bred an instinct for seeking to belong within a group (see Brewer 2007). Belonging is facilitated and communicated through nonverbal and verbal interpersonal interaction. Throughout the human lifespan, belonging and the constitutive interpersonal relating remain vital, as do the securing of fundamental necessary resources such as food and shelter. In Baumeister & Leary's (1995) research on the need to belong they concluded that this is a powerful, fundamental, and extremely pervasive motivation. There is a need for frequent, non-aversive interactions within an ongoing relational bond, and dissolution of existing bonds is resisted. Lack of attachments is linked to many ill effects on health, adjustment, and well-being. Another study showed with fMRI that being ostracised from a group activates the same region of the brain that is activated when physical pain is experienced (Eisenberger et al. 2003). And Van Beest & Williams (2006) demonstrated that even when experimental conditions are created whereby individuals receive monetary rewards when they are excluded by others in a game, being excluded still hurts. In other words, rejection always hurts – we all dread rejection.

Throughout life there are innumerable potentials for threats to security, whether in the form of threats to the person directly or to their protective other/s or their required resources, and evolution has selectively propagated humans who are most effectively alert to such potential threats so that danger to survival can best be averted. I view this alertness to threat as being what constitutes the propensity for anxiety that is endemic to the human condition, and I see the attempt to cope with and defend against such anxiety as being what has for all time fuelled the endeavours of religion, philosophy, psychology, politics, and industry. As Hollway & Jefferson (2013:21) have written in their definition of a person as a "psychosocial subject", each person is "a product of a unique biography of anxiety-provoking life-events and the manner in which [these] have been unconsciously defended against". They go on to say that "such defensive activities affect and are affected by discourses (systems of meaning that are a product of the social world)"; that such defences "are intersubjective processes (that is, they affect and are affected by others)"; and that "real events in the external, social world ... are discursively and defensively appropriated" (2013:21). I agree with Hollway & Jefferson (2013) that conceiving of persons in this way, as psychosocial subjects, is the conceptualisation that is most conducive to a serious engagement with researching human experience and behaviour.

In our ordinary course of life that is involved with seeking to meet the various goals described above, two major primary social phenomena are encountered: competition, and collaboration. Between members of any social group, and between groups, there is competition for the resources that exist at varying levels of scarcity and abundance at different points in time and circumstance, and there is the prospect of collaboration in order to help each other to secure such resources. I see the need to decide whether and when to compete against versus collaborate with another person as a primary quandary that at the most primitive level underlies all interpersonal relating. In other words, a constant (though not necessarily at all conscious) question is: are you my ally or my adversary?

Recognition: the interpersonal mirror that establishes self-esteem

It has been described above how infants are from birth relationally oriented, seeking to establish the most effective possible mutual bonds with caregivers. The fact that what these early interpersonal interactions and experiences are predominantly like for the child is highly formative of him or her is delineated by every major body of theory and knowledge that is concerned with human development and relationship, such as Attachment Theory, the Psychodynamic approach (including Object Relations), Humanistic (e.g. Person-Centred) approaches, Cognitive Behavioural Therapy, and Transactional Analysis. Relational psychoanalyst Jessica Benjamin (1995) argues that recognition is as important to psychological survival as food is to physical survival (cited in Hollway 2015:94). But what does recognition entail? For ease of reading, I will here refer to the caregiver as female and the infant as male.

Paediatrician, psychoanalyst, and Object Relations theorist Donald Winnicott (1965; 1975) explains in his developmental theory how an infant acquires his first sense of self through experiencing how another reacts to him. Winnicott named this process "mirroring": infants cry or smile, for example, and perceive from the reaction in their caregiver's eyes, facial expressions, posture, gestures, and volume, pitch and tone of voice, whether the caregiver is concerned or delighted, comfortable or uncomfortable, approving or disapproving. When a caregiver's reaction to an infant accurately mirrors back to the infant what his own experience is – for example smiling appreciatively at the infant's enjoyment or showing solicitous concern at his distress – the infant feels acknowledged and validated. In this way the infant's inner experience becomes "joined up" with the exterior world through a matrix of interpersonal interaction and the infant feels "real" (Winnicott 1971; 1975). That this is how early interpersonal development proceeds has all since been confirmed by neuropsychological research (see Schore 2016). If an infant experiences the benefit of predominantly accurate mirroring, with neither neglect nor impingement from the caregiver, and experiences the caregiver showing in her responses that she is accepting of the infant's full range of expressiveness – not being unduly alarmed by manifestations of the infant's various states, and neither collapsing nor retaliating in the face of extreme states in the infant – then the infant develops what Winnicott termed his "True Self" (Winnicott 1960). Infants soon learn which kinds of expressiveness are discouraged or even punished by their caregivers, and begin to shut down the expressiveness of emotions, behaviours, and later desires, questions, opinions, and thoughts that meet with an unfavourable response. All of us are so sensitive to these cues because of their importance in constituting our security which is linked with ensuring our survival.

Many of these early interpersonal experiences occur before a person has developed the faculties for symbolising such experiences in language and accessing them in conscious memory that can be verbally articulated. However, they have a pervasive impact. How this can play out specifically where a very high-IQ individual is involved, and the intrapersonal and interpersonal effects, is detailed in the next chapter (Chapter 4, "Recognition and reactions"). But what specific characteristics are associated with very high IQ?

Person: the extremely high-IQ individual

The defining of extreme intelligence by means of an IQ score of 130 and higher, i.e. 98th percentile and above, has been explained in the Introduction. However, outside of IQ score, how might extreme intelligence manifest and be identified?

As described, the concept of giftedness overlaps with that of extreme intelligence, and there are numerous different conceptions of what giftedness entails (e.g. see Sternberg & Davidson 2005). In the literature on intelligence and giftedness I see three main dimensions to this: a biological basis, related experiential and behavioural characteristics, and minority status.

Biological basis

As Chapter 2 has shown, extreme intelligence has been evidenced to have a biological basis that is largely genetically determined and involves an atypical neurological profile (see the subsection "What produces intelligence?"). A study of 3,715 American Mensa members showed that as well as having elevated intellectual capacity ("hyper brain"), this sample also had elevated sensory, immune, and inflammatory responses ("hyper body") (Karpinski et al. 2018).

Experiential and behavioural characteristics

These biological differences give rise to associated experiential and behavioural characteristics. Speed and efficiency in learning and performing other cognitive tasks is a hallmark feature of high IQ/giftedness (Saccuzzo et al. 1994). However, extending beyond cognitive performance, in 1964 Polish psychologist Kazimierz Dabrowski identified five areas of "overexcitability" or "supersensitivity" associated with giftedness: psychomotor, sensual, emotional, intellectual, and imaginational (Daniels & Piechowski 2009). These manifest as heightened intensity, sensitivity, excitability, perceptiveness, complexity, energy, and drive in each of those five areas. In 1978 Joseph Renzulli added to this the importance of behavioural characteristics of gifted individuals, identified as high levels of task commitment (motivation) and creativity (Renzulli 1978). A new significant contribution was made by the Columbus Group in 1991 (cited in Silverman 2013), who conceptualised giftedness as asynchronous development. This refers to the uneven development seen in gifted children where their advanced cognitive functioning can be far ahead of their chronological age, yet their emotional maturation is not advanced and can even lag behind that expected for their chronological age. They might also reach developmental stages earlier, and more intensely, than is the norm (Webb et al. 2016). Another characteristic of highly intelligent individuals has been termed multipotentiality (Webb et al. 2016; Daniels & Piechowski 2009). This refers to what is often their capacity to do many things well, evidencing high potential in many different directions simultaneously. This is what we see in individuals who become polymaths.

Minority status

This third dimension of minority status relates to the fact that extreme intelligence or giftedness occurs in a small minority of people worldwide (Freeman 2005). How it is perceived, identified, and responded to varies significantly in different countries and cultures around the world (Freeman 2016; Grobman 2017a). However, it always involves being statistically an extreme deviation from the norm (Nauta & Ronner 2013:3; Silverman 2013). What this means is that it causes very high-IQ individuals to stand out from their peers in how they behave, how they perform on tasks, how they are perceived by others, and how they feel about themselves (Silverman 2013).

When asked what they saw as constituting their high IQ, my research interviewees made quantitative comparisons of their performance with that of others (noticing that they would achieve more than others could in the same amount of time, such as: speed of seeing solutions; deeper, better, and faster understanding; and number of different aspects perceived), and they made qualitative comments about having a passion to always be learning, and an enjoyment of and need to keep busy with challenges such as solving problems. I formed the most frequently mentioned qualities into three main categories: way of perceiving the

TABLE 3.1 Manifestations of very high IQ

Way of perceiving the world (Corresponds with biological basis)	Way of engaging with the world (Corresponds with the associated experiential and behavioural characteristics)	Performance relative to that of others (Corresponds with minority status)
• Quickly sees solutions. • Capacity for seeing the whole picture, seeing patterns, and thinking strategically. • Sees a lot of different aspects to everything. • Creative thinker.	• Enjoyment of and need for keeping busy with challenges, such as solving problems. • Passion to always be learning. • Loves reading. • High confidence in own ability to do anything.	• Deeper, better, faster understanding than others. • Found school very easy. • Has had an identity of being best at things. • Special facility for language (good with words and spelling) and/or maths. • Speaks fast. • Started reading very young. • Original thinker.

world, way of engaging with the world, and performance relative to that of others. It can be seen that these three categories correspond, respectively, with the three dimensions detailed above of biological basis, associated experiential and behavioural characteristics, and minority status (see Table 3.1). So, for example, I grouped a love of reading within the category of "way of engaging with the world", but placed the fact of having learned to read at a very young age into the category of "performance relative to others".

Extreme intelligence "pervasively affects" (Webb et al. 2016:257) a person's life: giftedness is a "quantitatively, qualitatively, and motivationally different way of experiencing life" (Jacobsen 2008:19). Sixteen of my interviewees were asked to rate on a scale of 1–10 how important giftedness was in their personal identity. Fourteen of the 16 chose the high end of the scale, from 7 to 10. More than half went as high as the highest rankings, 9 or 10:

> At least 8–9 … I think I'd say it was 8 or 9 because the simple fact is that anyone who knows me will see eventually that is a major part of my personality, having to understand things, having to explain things, and not just sitting there and agreeing with everything I'm told, especially when I know it's wrong.
>
> *(Wayne)*

Let's say 8 because there is a freedom in knowing that, or at least assuming that, you can learn anything that you want to learn, so if you have an interest or you're fascinated by something, you can learn it.

(Erik)

When the key high-IQ features of having the ability to learn fast and the associated drive to be regularly learning – what Meier et al. (2014) identified as a "need for cognition", and Winner (2012) termed a "rage to master" – are engaged with and satisfied, the individual feels happy and fulfilled. When such abilities are not engaged with and are frustrated and wasted, the individual is unhappy and can develop low self-esteem and mental health problems ranging from mild depression through to suicidality (Falck 2013).

Goals revisited

Although a high-IQ individual will share with all other human beings the same survival-related goals delineated above, his or her personal goals might differ somewhat from those of people who do not have very high IQ. Evolutionary psychology accepts that humans have not changed very much since the end of the Pleistocene epoch about 10,000 years ago, meaning that we evolved in adaptation to living in the African savanna as hunter-gatherers in small bands of 50 or so related individuals, and this is what is termed our ancestral environment (Kanazawa 2004). Kanazawa (2004) coined the term Savanna Principle to denote that human behaviour is based on conditions and assumptions forged in this ancestral environment. Kanazawa (2012) argues that extreme intelligence is an evolutionary anomaly because it is not something that was needed for general survival in the constancy and continuity of the ancestral environment, but which evolved to deal with occasionally emerging novel, nonrecurrent problems.

According to this, an extremely intelligent person is different from the norm in that the usual evolutionary goals of subsistence and reproduction, which are satisfying to the majority of people, are not what motivates those with high IQ, who gravitate instead towards novelty and seek complex and challenging problems to solve. Kanazawa (2012) presents many different domains of behaviour in which highly intelligent individuals have been shown to have different preferences (including in religion, musical tastes, and political affiliations) from those with average IQ. These differences involve a preference for the uncommon – such as preferences for atheism, classical music, and liberalism (and studying for PhDs), which are all recent and novel developments in the history of humankind. Extremely intelligent individuals' needs to utilise their abilities, and their apparent focus on achievement goals in priority over affiliation goals, could be said to reflect their purpose as serving the community by being on the periphery of it attending to unusual problems rather than being in the midst of it focused on ordinary daily life. An example of this is a very high-IQ client of mine who talks of wanting to live a life not focused on collecting subjective experiences like memorable holidays, but one focused on making an objective difference in the world that will outlast her own lifespan. A key lens through which she approaches her life is, "What will be written on my tombstone?"

Extremely high IQ is a condition that is distinct from any of its potential outcomes. Outcomes vary greatly according to how its characteristics are responded to, which brings us to the impact of the environment in which the extremely intelligent person finds him- or herself.

Environment: country, culture, family, school, workplace

Every person's interpersonal environment is made up of the macrocosm of a particular country and culture, and microcosms of particular social groups within structures such as family, school, and workplace. Such environments can differ substantially in how they respond to individuals' manifestations of extreme intelligence. This was evident from my research interviewees: they originated from several different countries; many had also moved between different countries, schools or workplaces; and they often drew comparisons between the different environments they had experienced. The experiences they described are also products of the particular time in history at which they occurred, influenced by, for example, that specific period's prevailing political regimes or educational policies. In presenting such material, I additionally see the environments (countries, cultures, families, etc.) of which my interviewees spoke not as objectively existing entities that were being reliably described, but as constructions that are contributed to by many personal factors including the selectivity of memory. I therefore see each environment described as an "environment in the mind" (inspired by Armstrong's (2004) notion of "the organisation in the mind"). Such environments do, however, always also have some basis in objective reality, and the experiences they provoked invariably produced longstanding impact on self-esteem, expectations, and behaviour.

Person–environment reciprocal recognition and interaction

In thinking about person–environment interaction a great number of factors are involved including gender, ethnicity, and SES. We will encounter examples of effects of these variables, but my focus is specifically on the variable of extreme intelligence and how characteristics associated with this affect person–environment reciprocal recognition and interaction. It is apparent from my research that no matter what kind of environment the high-IQ child finds him- or herself in, that environment will come to recognise in the child the manifestations of extreme intelligence – whether or not these are labelled as such – and will react to this in some way. And what I found is that the single most important basic point about the environments that high-IQ individuals find themselves in, is whether such environments are benign, supportive, welcoming, and encouraging towards or even valuing of manifestations of high ability and able to engage with these, or not. For example, in adult life job satisfaction was highest for interviewees who had mentioned having a work environment that was in this manner conducive (Falck 2013).

The first persons that newborn infants usually come into regular close contact with are their parents and the other members of their family of origin, so these are the people that form their first social environment and who respond in one way or another to the nature of the child they are beginning to experience. After this first family-of-origin environment, usually the next social environment that a child is most regularly exposed to and therefore most influenced by is that of the school/s he or she attends. Family environments can differ markedly in how they respond to the characteristics of a high-IQ child. Some interviewees experienced a strong discouragement of manifestations of high IQ, even to the extent of being regularly physically beaten for expressing precocious curiosity and eloquence. John, who grew up in England, explained:

> I was out of line over and over and over again. I had opinions and I articulated them and I insisted on coming back to them and even after he [his father] might have told me to shut up or he'd make me shut up, I would just keep going and keep going and keep going ... He was just trying to crush me. I mean he was just trying to make me shut up and toe the line ...

The latter is something that was also experienced growing up in other countries, such as was described by Avi from India:

> In my own family I was bullied big time, especially by my father, yes. So he felt intellectually threatened ... definitely 'til 11 I used to get beaten big time by my father. And if I said something very sharp or, for example, if he asked me a response to ... a simple example would be like two plus two is four, but then hey, one-and-a-half and two-and-a-half is also four, do you see what I mean? So I was able to think out of the box and come up with different kinds of solutions, but if that was not the answer he was expecting he would beat me up. So that was really horrible and I hated him all the way.

In contrast, Gill, who, like John, also grew up in England, was encouraged so much in her high-IQ qualities that she did her GCSE exams a full three years early, at the age of 13: "some of the time I felt I was also being a bit too pushed, it was a lot of, 'You have to do this, you have to do well'".

In comparing the environments experienced in different countries, a main comparison that was made was between the Eastern Bloc countries of Eastern

Germany and Russia, and Western European countries. The former were described as having a culture where "you don't show yourself" (Ana). Ana described how Russian and East German culture "pushed her down" so much – "it's a big suffering" – that when she came on a trip to London where this was not the case she decided "I need to move there". Hans, who grew up in East Germany and then moved to West Germany at the age of 15, described a "very, very competitive" boy who was in his class in West Germany: "Never met such a person before in East Germany, 'cos they wouldn't exist". In this new school in this new country, he experienced that – after a culture where "I almost tried to hide that I knew more than the teacher" – everything had changed: "Now suddenly, I was in an environment group that was very much encouraged to know more, to be better"; there was "suddenly no holding back".

Gill, like Hans, also had very different experiences of school, this time not because they were in different countries (both of her schools were in England) but based on whether it was a school environment that promoted intellectual accomplishment or did not support it. She described having had "a very rocky up and down time" at school:

> I suppose the comprehensive school that I went to, I did definitely get, I wouldn't go so far as to say I was bullied but I got teased for achieving well and I certainly felt I needed to dumb myself down to fit in more …

She then went to a grammar school (involving selective entry based on academic competence) which was "a lot easier, I felt much happier there, it did make a difference". In this environment achieving well was required and esteemed, and Gill no longer had to disguise her capability and love of learning.

Two interviewees described Scandinavian societies as egalitarian, where "people are expected to be equal" (Max, speaking about Sweden) and "when you just turn up in a normal class there and you perform very well … then people might … treat you a bit badly". Hans described how in West Germany, the UK, and the USA he experienced needing to write "the CV, the resume" in a way that is "all about my fantastic achievements", whereas in Denmark after his CV written in that style was read at a job interview he was told: "You're quite a show off".

Mei, from Hong Kong, compared personal with workplace environments, and introduced a gender angle. She described how she had to be careful not to "too much out-perform" her husband in family and social contexts because Chinese culture required a female to "respect your husband more being head of the family and so on". Within her professional context in London, however, she could "absolutely be myself". London was repeatedly described as a place that was valued for offering great diversity and freedom:

> It's brilliant … yeah … I mean, I love it. I wish it worked like this everywhere. London is particularly special in that respect.
>
> *(Hans)*

Although several interviewees had moved from other countries to be in the UK, and almost idealised London where they were now based, there were British-born interviewees who spoke of wider British culture in more strictured terms:

> Brits don't like putting themselves forward or being better, there's this natural reservedness about British people that says don't stand out, don't celebrate achievement in many ways.
>
> *(Tracy)*

> The average person, especially the average British person, mocks intelligence.
>
> *(Jane)*

Moving between environments: transferring habits and expectations

Through all these experiences of the person and environment interacting with each other, the high-IQ individual is learning from the interactions, and based on these experiences is forming habits and expectations. For example, take this quote from interviewee Tess about her transition from school to university:

> I found it baffling that there were intelligent people there who were also, you know, socially brilliant and wonderful and everyone wanted to be around them and I was like, but you're clever. You know. So I found that ... you know, I found it really hard, really hard.
>
> *(Tess)*

Until her arrival at university she had experienced her intelligence as not being welcomed, and had formed a strong association between being "clever" and being socially undesirable. Having to now re-evaluate that association was something she found "baffling" and "really hard" to have to adapt to. She recognised that the school environment she had experienced was different from other kinds of school environments. She said of a colleague:

> He went to a very good school full of similar people and yeah ... you know at those schools it was cool to be intelligent. At my school ... in a sort of like village comprehensive with, you know, real mixed ability, a variety of levels, it was not cool to be clever.
>
> *(Tess)*

Here she has formed expectations based on her experiences in one environment – i.e. "it was not cool to be clever" – and then carried that expectation over to other environments, such as university, for which it was not apt.

64   Development

A similar experience was reported by other interviewees also, of having formed habits in one environment which they might then inappropriately apply in a different environment. A common experience of this involved high-IQ individuals in under-stimulating environments forming habits of laziness, which would then not prepare them for the increased effort required of them for success in more demanding environments (this is discussed further in Chapter 4). As Gill said:

> I think it is something that in the past I have possibly been complacent with and thought, "Oh I'll do well in this without doing any work", which isn't always the case obviously.

Erik described how he was "caught off-guard" when he started going about in his habitual way within a new work environment that was highly selective and how he was surprised by the differences he encountered:

> At previous workplaces, it seems like I had more time, certainly more time than now, but I had more time than the average person. In that time people would ask me things, how this or that worked, and that was interesting to explain so you became, I was like an oracle for things, so achieving less than I do now … but explaining more because now I don't have to explain things because people know. Either they know it or it's much quicker for other people to understand things, to the point where people have caught me off-guard. I just do a couple of words and they're quicker than you think they'd be able to understand the sentence, they reply and you're, "Wait – that's completely right!" It was almost like they replied so quickly you didn't think it was a serious answer. So I have to explain things a lot less now.

High-IQ individuals experiencing themselves as being good at things, perhaps particularly without much effort being required, and this being noticed by others, sometimes with the result of gaining an identity as the person who is best at something – "an oracle" – can create in such persons a sense of unswerving confidence in their own ability:

> I'm very particular and very pushy about how something has to be done, because I have this unfailing belief – which is a fault of mine, I must admit – that my way is the best way or the right way, and occasionally other people will say "Oh he's very sure that this is right, he's very confident".
>
> *(Wayne)*

In this excerpt Wayne cites this attitude of his as a fault. His regular experience at school, described earlier in his interview, of getting the answers "all right" and "being good at passing exams", appears to have set up for him a firm belief in being right. Perhaps he now sees this as a fault because it has continued into situations where he has come to experience that he has not been right. However, he might also be seeing it as a fault as a consequence of feedback from the environment that has led him to realise that others find such behaviour objectionable. As interviewee Don said, "Nobody wants to be around somebody [who's] every time right".

The kinds of parenting, schooling, and workplace practices represented here and their effects will be further discussed in Chapter 9. But what this section has done is give a taste of the different kinds of environments high-IQ individuals can find themselves in and how much these can differ according to whether the individual's manifestation of high ability is welcomed and even encouraged, or frowned upon and even violently deterred. It has also shown how person–environment interaction leads to learning from experience and to the forming of habits and expectations, and that these might then be transferred from one environment to another for which they are not always appropriate.

Three kinds of change

In general, if any organism is achieving its goals there will be no reason to effect change to the status quo, as change requires endeavour, and a general principle of conserving energy and resources means that change will not be entered into without a convincingly motivating rationale. What became apparent from my research interviews was that it was often the negative effects of experiencing interpersonal difficulty (such as problems in a workplace) or negative mental health effects that provided the catalyst for seeking to modify some aspect of the status quo to try to bring about improvement.

I saw within my research data three main ways that interviewees had been involved in trying to make changes so as to improve the outcomes they were experiencing (see Figure 3.2). The first kind of change involved trying to make a change to their own nature; the second involved making a change to the nature of their environment by moving to a different environment. The third kind of change related to working on the interface between the person and the environment: trying to change their way of interacting with their environment could bring about a different response from the environment.

The first kind of change involves high-IQ persons trying to change who they are by, for example – as Gill described above – trying to "dumb themselves down", or even relinquishing their (unpopular) interests and suppressing their "rage to master". However, whilst a person's nature can be hidden, or disavowed, it cannot be fundamentally changed. The price of attempting such change is usually paid in deteriorating mental health.

The second kind of change is represented in many examples above of interviewees moving to different countries, schools, or workplaces, and how that could make a big difference to what was expected of them, the sorts of

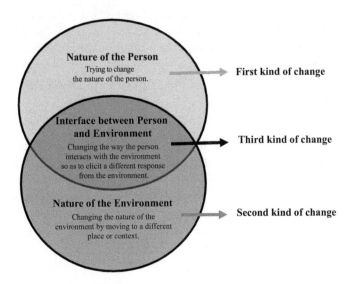

FIGURE 3.2 Three kinds of change

responses they received, and the experiences and outcomes that ensued. Here again, I say this is something that "could" make a big difference, because if a person has had problems and carries on behaving as they always have but just in a different environment, it is not certain that they will not simply experience the same problems again in the new environment. Examples of this are apparent in the trajectories of high-IQ individuals who move from job to job and even from dismissal to dismissal (Nauta & Corten 2002). It might also be that moving to a different environment is not possible.

The third kind of change does not do violence to the nature of the person, nor does it make improvement dependant on a move to a different environment. Also, with an improvement in a person's way of interacting with their environment, even when a move to a different environment might be helpful and has been undertaken, it minimises the risk that the same old problems will simply recur in the new environment. This is discussed further in Chapter 9, "Helping high ability thrive".

Summary

This chapter has situated extreme intelligence within a wider framework of mainstream psychological theory. An evolutionary perspective, Attachment Theory, the neuroscience of intersubjectivity, and major Humanistic and Psychodynamic theories have been drawn on to show that our biopsychosocial lifespan development is shaped by a need for security that is expressed in an essential search for relationship from infancy onwards and a primitive survivalist alertness to safety and danger (alerting us to the danger of extremes). Safety involves being noticed, recognised, being taken care of and belonging, and danger is being rejected, abandoned, and not having the resources (including material and social) that are needed for survival. An original "High-IQ Context" model has been presented that gives an overview of how these core issues combine. Excerpts from my research interviews have been presented to show how high-IQ individuals seek to fulfil these needs to be noticed, to belong, to collaborate and to compete – dreading the pain and danger of rejection – within environments that can differ markedly as to how much acceptance, understanding, or support they provide for such individuals. Characteristics associated with high IQ/giftedness have been analysed, and an original change model derived from my research data has been presented. Foundational concepts that have been introduced include self-actualisation (Maslow); mirroring (Winnicott); the attachment system and internal working model (Bowlby); and True Self (Winnicott).

References

Ainsworth, M. D., Blehar, M. C., Waters, E. & Wall, S. (1978). *Patterns of Attachment: A Psychological Study of the Strange Situation*. Hillsdale, NJ: Erlbaum.

Armstrong, D. (2004). *Organisation in the Mind: Psychoanalysis, Group Relations and Organisational Consultancy*. The Tavistock Clinic Series, edited by R. French. London: Karnac Books.

Bartholomew, K. & Horowitz, L. M. (1991). Attachment styles among young adults: A test of a four-category model. *Journal of Personality and Social Psychology*, 61, pp. 226–244.

Baumeister, R. F. & Leary, M. R. (1995). The need to belong: desire for interpersonal attachments as a fundamental human motivation. *Psychological Bulletin*, 117, pp. 497–529.

Benjamin, J. (1995). *Like Subjects, Love Objects*. New Haven, CT: Yale University Press.

Bowlby, J. (1969). *Attachment and Loss: Vol.1, Attachment*. New York: Basic Books.

Bowlby, J. (1973). *Attachment and Loss: Vol.2, Separation, Anxiety and Anger*. New York: Basic Books.

Bowlby, J. (1980). *Attachment and Loss: Vol.3, Loss*. New York: Basic Books.

Bowlby, J. (1988). *A Secure Base*. London: Routledge.

Bowlby, J., Robertson, J. & Rosenbluth, D. (1952). A two-year old goes to hospital. *The Psychoanalytic Study of the Child*, 7, pp. 82–84.

Brewer, M. B. (2007). The importance of being we: human nature and intergroup relations. *American Psychologist*, 62(8), pp. 728–738.

Cannon, W. B. (1939). *The Wisdom of the Body*. New York: Norton.

Daniels, S. & Piechowski, M. M. (Eds.). (2009). *Living with Intensity*. Tucson, AZ: Great Potential Press.

Eisenberger, N. I., Lieberman, M. D. & Williams, K. D. (2003). Does rejection hurt? An fMRI study of social exclusion. *Science*, 302, pp. 290–292.

Erikson, E. H. (1950). *Childhood and Society*. New York: W. W. Norton & Company.

Falck, S. (2013). *Attachment Styles and Experience of Workplace Interpersonal Relating in Intellectually Gifted Adults*. Unpublished Practice Evaluation Project (PEP) submitted in partial fulfilment of the requirements for the Doctorate in Psychotherapy by Professional Studies at Metanoia Institute/Middlesex University.

Freeman, J. (2005). Permission to be gifted: how conceptions of giftedness can change lives. In: R. J. Sternberg & J. E. Davidson (Eds.). *Conceptions of Giftedness*. (2nd ed.). Cambridge: Cambridge University Press. pp. 80–97.

Freeman, J. (2016). *Academic Consultation Meeting*. [Discussion] (Personal communication, 23 September 2016).

Gerhardt, S. (2015). *Why Love Matters*. (2nd ed.). New York: Routledge.

Grobman, J. (2017a). *Academic Consultation Meeting*. [Phonecall] (Personal communication, 19 March 2017).

Harris, W. V. (1994). Child-exposure in the Roman Empire. *The Journal of Roman Studies*, 84, pp. 1–22.

Hazan, C. & Shaver, P. (1987). Romantic love conceptualized as an attachment process. *Journal of Personality and Social Psychology*, 52, pp. 511–524.

Hollway, W. (2015). *Knowing Mothers: Researching Maternal Identity Change. Studies in the Psychosocial*. London: Palgrave Macmillan.

Hollway, W. & Jefferson, T. (2013). *Doing Qualitative Research Differently – A Psychosocial Approach*. (2nd ed.). London: Sage.

Howe, D. (2011). *Attachment Across the Lifecourse*. New York: Palgrave Macmillan.

Jacobsen, M.-E. (2008). Giftedness in the workplace: can the bright mind thrive in today's organizations? *Mensa Research Journal*, 39(2), pp. 15–20.

Kanazawa, S. (2004). The Savanna Principle. *Managerial and Decision Economics*, 25, pp. 41–54.

Kanazawa, S. (2012). *The Intelligence Paradox*. Hoboken, NJ: John Wiley & Sons.

Karpinski, R. I., Kinase Kolb, A. M., Tetreault, N. A. & Borowski, T. B. (2018). High intelligence: a risk factor for psychological and physiological overexcitabilities. *Intelligence*, 66, pp. 8–23.

Maslow, A. H. (1943). A theory of human motivation. *Psychological Review*, 50(4), pp. 370–396.

Meier, E., Vogl, K. & Preckel, F. (2014). Motivational characteristics of students in gifted classes: the pivotal role of need for cognition. *Learning and Individual Differences*, 33, pp. 39–46.

Nauta, N. & Corten, F. (2002). Gifted adults in work (English translation). *Tijdschrift voor Bedrijfs- en Verzekeringsgeneeeskunde* (Journal for Occupational and Insurance Physicians), 10(11), pp. 332–335. [online] Available at: www.sengifted.org/archives/articles/gifted-adults-in-work. [Accessed 12 June 2012].

Nauta, N. & Ronner, S. (2013). *Gifted Workers Hitting the Target*. The Netherlands: Shaker Media.

Renzulli, J. S. (1978). What makes giftedness? Reexamining a definition. *Phi Delta Kappan*, 60, pp. 180–184.

Saccuzzo, D. P., Johnson, N. E. & Guertin, T. L. (1994). Information processing in gifted versus nongifted African American, Latino, Filipino, and White children: speeded versus nonspeeded paradigms. *Intelligence*, 19(2), pp. 219–243.

Schore, A. N. (2016). *Affect Regulation and the Origin of the Self*. New York: Routledge.

Silverman, L. K. (2013). *Giftedness 101*. New York: Springer Publishing Company.

Sroufe, L. A. (1989). Relationships, self and individual adaptation. In: A. Samerof & R. Emde (Eds.). *Relationship Disturbances in Childhood*. New York: Basic Books. pp. 70–94.

Stern, D. N. (1985). *The Interpersonal World of the Infant: A View from Psychoanalysis and Developmental Psychology*. New York: Basic Books.

Sternberg, R. J. & Davidson, J. E. (Eds.). (2005). *Conceptions of Giftedness*. (2nd ed.). Cambridge: Cambridge University Press.

Van Beest, I. & Williams, K. D. (2006). When inclusion costs and ostracism pays, ostracism still hurts. *Journal of Personality and Social Psychology*, 91, pp. 918–928.

Webb, J. T., Amend, E. R., Beljan, P., Webb, N. E., Kuzujanakis, M., Olenchak, F. R. & Goerss, J. (2016). *Misdiagnosis and Dual Diagnoses of Gifted Children and Adults*. (2nd ed.). Tucson, AZ: Great Potential Press.

Winberg, J. (2005). Mother and newborn baby: mutual regulation of physiology and behavior – A selective review. *Developmental Psychobiology*, 47(3), pp. 217–229.

Winner, E. (2012). Gifted Children. In: *ParentEdge*. pp. 75–81. [online] Available at: www.gifted.gr/documents/useful-documents/Gifted_children.pdf. [Accessed 3 March 2019].

Winnicott, D. W. (1960). Ego distortion in terms of true and false self. In: D. W. Winnicott (Ed.). *The Maturational Processes and the Facilitating Environment*. Reprint 1990. London: Karnac Books. pp. 140–152.

Winnicott, D. W. (1965). *The Maturational Processes and the Facilitating Environment*. Reprint 2005. London: Karnac Books.

Winnicott, D. W. (1971). *Playing and Reality*. New York: Routledge Classics.

Winnicott, D. W. (1975). *Collected Papers: Through Paediatrics to Psycho-Analysis*. London: Tavistock Publications.

PART II
Predicaments

4

RECOGNITION AND REACTIONS

What happens when someone stands out so much?

> **Reflective Prompt 4:** Can you think of a memorable experience you have had of noticing that someone else seemed to have a very different level of ability (higher or lower) compared with your own? In what circumstances did this become apparent? What thoughts and feelings did this stir in you about that person? What thoughts and feelings did this stir in you about yourself? After you noticed this, did it change the way you behaved towards that person? How?

We have covered (in Chapter 2) how it is that some people come to stand out so much from others: now we examine how people react when they encounter a person who stands out in this way. And how is such a person affected by the recognition of being extremely capable? The current chapter also links with the previous chapter by showing how the consequences of standing out from others relate to the core issues outlined there. For example, standing out brings about an exaggeration of being noticed or recognised, which can be a fantasised ideal. This relates to safety, such as how a leader in a group can have the security of being the most valued member of the group with access to the most resources. But standing out also involves being "set apart", identified as different, and can produce the consequence of feeling that you don't fit in, don't belong, and are isolated. This relates to danger, such as a leader also being especially visible and therefore vulnerable to being conspicuously devalued, ousted, even assassinated. To explore this we will start at the very beginning of life.

Comparing and competing

A baby is born. "Every child is a gift", as people commonly say, or "a gift from God" as the original biblical reference puts it (Psalm 127:3). As Freud (1914:91) famously put it, we are born "His Majesty the Baby", commanding the rapt attention of those close to us who attend to our every need. At first, every little thing we do is greeted by our parents as phenomenally interesting and brilliant. But as Kaufman (2008) writes, every child is a gift and every child has gifts, but not every child is gifted according to the definition of what giftedness is. Soon comparison – what Theodore Roosevelt (n.d.) termed "the thief of joy" – sets in. People compare their babies with each other: they check which one has reached which developmental milestone, being worried if their baby seems delayed, feeling proud if their baby seems advanced. Right from the beginning of life there are sets of developmental yardsticks (e.g. in Sharma & Cockerill 2014) that establish what the norm is for things such as when babies are meant to have gained a certain weight or used their first two-word phrase, and parents and health professionals measure growing infants against these. Partly this is about checking for developmental problems that might require intervention, but on a more visceral level for parents this comparing is driven by a fear of their child being delayed as this could mean being left out, "left behind", when staying within the group is what is safest. But there is also satisfaction and pride if their child is advanced because that is reassuring of the prospect of being able to successfully compete.

Being able to compete successfully can lead to a more secure place in a group, even becoming the leader of a group, and being the leader is associated with high status and lower levels of stress (Sherman et al. 2012). In human and animal groups there is generally a hierarchy of positions of varying status, and high status amasses certain advantages (see Magee & Galinsky 2009). With hens there is the exemplar pecking order. In primates, the species most similar to our own, individuals with higher status in the troop often have less stress, better health, more success in accessing food supplies and in mating, and live longer (Sapolsky 2005). Within human evolution too, higher hierarchical positions have been associated with better health and longevity (Wilkinson 2001). Higher positions of this kind in contemporary Western society are most commonly gained by securing professional careers, therefore successfully passing the selection procedures that give admission to such careers is valued. However, as mentioned in Chapter 1 (and which will be elaborated on in Chapter 6), it is IQs near the top of the normal range that are most correlated with success of this kind. What seems to be most desired therefore is to avoid extremes and be safely within the norms of the group, yet just ahead enough to ensure the best survival prospects for yourself and your offspring. That is what parents are checking for by comparing their children with each other (though they are very unlikely to be consciously formulating or expressing that this is what they mean to be doing).

When the children start school, they themselves engage in comparing. In Erikson's (1950) life-stages model, for school-aged children prior to adolescence (i.e. aged 5–12 years) he names the psychosocial crisis that has to be navigated as "industry versus inferiority", and cites the virtue that is gained through mastery of this stage as being that of competence. The developing child derives his own sense of competence by comparing and measuring his performance against that of others (Eccles 1999), and by comparing the way his performance is responded to with the way others' performances are responded to (Erikson 1968). According to this, comparison is an inevitable component of seeking to build self-esteem.

Children at school quickly pick out and label as "clever" those who do best – the child who drew the best picture, or knew the most answers, or was quickest at completing a task. Status is accorded to this. In this way it is registered who is likely to prove to be either the most formidable adversary, or, with their admired competence, the most confidence-inspiring potential ally. What comes to be judged "the best" is also bound up with noticing what reaction their respective efforts have produced: who got the most praise? The highest grades? There is a naturally inbuilt competitiveness to gain approval because having the caregiver's favour and attention ensures survival by being kept in mind, protected, provided for, and not at risk of being neglected or abandoned. And because of that competitiveness, there is a fine line between admiration and denigration: those who have a position of status can also be resented and attract attempts to destroy their advantage (overt envious attacks) or at the least stimulate pleasure being taken in any misfortune they should suffer (the more insidious *Schadenfreude*).

Being recognised by others

As mentioned in the previous chapter, whatever environment the very high-IQ child is in, manifestations of his or her unusual intelligence will in some way be recognised, even if not labelled as such, and will be reacted to in some way: there is a moment, or event, of recognition, or a series of these. Such recognition could be informal, for example:

> It was sort of identified early on, oh, you know, you're intelligent. You're not so good at sports ... Like no one sort of said, "Hey [Sean], you know, do you wanna go up for the football team or the baseball team?" But they did say, "Hey [Sean], do you wanna join the chess team or the debate team?"
>
> *(Sean)*

Or such recognition could be formal, for example:

> What happened eventually, when I was about eight or nine I got taken in the office one day after my latest bout of misbehaviour. I was in the office

with one of the senior teachers, this was in England, and I was introduced to a gentleman, I remember his name actually, it was Dr [name]. I actually remember his name. This is going back into the 70s. My dad came up the school, he was there, with Dr [name], the teacher and me, and I got these tests to do. They asked me [questions] … And … they all looked at each other and nodded and smiled and they carried on with more questions, and I had questions about probability, like playing cards. I didn't know anything about cards at that age so they explained to me what a pack of cards was, so I worked the answers out and got them all right. That was it. About half an hour later I went back to class and my dad went home. Later that evening I'd come home from school, my dad came home from work … I said, "What was all this about, what were these questions about at school?", and he said to me, "I've got a genius", and he laughed. That's all I knew … It must have been an IQ test. Obviously the teachers had become concerned about me and they'd obviously explained to someone I messed around a lot at school but I was very clever, so obviously they set up a test for me …

(Wayne)

The recognition and reaction that comes is rarely neutral. At the two extremes, it can be positive (rewarding), such as receiving affirmation/validation, compliments, approval, praise, awards, popularity, and later in life securing desired jobs, promotions, and remuneration packages. Or it can be negative (punishing), for example being clashed with, disapproved of, rejected, excluded, blocked. Several interviewees reported having been bullied at school for achieving well. In the example above, the positive smiles and nods are noticed by the child and remembered decades later. Yermish (2010:16) states that:

> A person's self-concept can be construed as the sum of all of their own beliefs about their status, including traits, social roles, relationships, and the like, and is built upon the accreditations and degradations they have experienced.

She draws on Garfinkel (1956), Schwartz (1979), and Ossorio (2006) in explaining that "accreditation and degradation ceremonies" (Yermish 2010:16) involve three players – someone who has some personal characteristic or performs some behaviour; someone who reacts to this in some way, who is seen as a member in good standing in a shared community of people; and someone who witnesses this reaction taking place. The playing out of this event is termed a ceremony, where the reaction of the "member in good standing" as observed by a witness results in the person who is being reacted to being either accredited (assigned a better status within the community) or degraded (assigned a worse status within the community). In the ordinary course of daily life growing up, an extremely intelligent person will experience a series of accreditations or degradations, building their self-concept and sense of whether or how much they are approved of and belong within the community or interpersonal environment in which they find themselves.

Most of my interviewees described school as being the context in which they remembered their high ability as having first been recognised by others. Whether the way it was recognised accorded accreditation or degradation is, however, not always clear-cut, as the incidents involved could be quite nuanced or multi-layered. For example, Mei described her chemistry teacher saying to her "You're just too brilliant, I can't find a question that you can't answer." But he also said "Why do you need to be so good in chemistry? You'll just end up in the kitchen anyway". A schoolteacher counts as a member in good standing in the community, and the witnesses to this teacher's reaction to Mei would be the other children in the classroom. But would the teacher's reaction here constitute a ceremony of accreditation or of degradation? He is complimenting her – "you're brilliant" – which constitutes accreditation. But there is another message in there: this is not actually what is required/desired within this community; as a Chinese female your real place is in the kitchen. What she's being told is that what she's exhibiting therefore is irrelevant or inappropriate/useless – you are "too" brilliant. This constitutes degradation.

For several interviewees, recognition of their extreme intelligence by others came in the form of standing out during regular school rituals that typically involved levels of attainment, perhaps set up as a competition, and the high-IQ individual would get to the top in unexpectedly rapid time and then stay at the top, sometimes in a band all on their own, with nowhere further to go. Tess described:

> We had like, it was like a spelling thing and you had different levels and they were all different colours of the rainbow. And so red level was very low and then I was the only one on violet, which was the last level.

She was on her own in that highest group for several years until a new boy joined the school who was placed at the same level with her. Consequences of this sort of situation would be the high-ability individual feeling bored (Helene: "School was ... an unmitigated hell ...", "intellectually it was a dead zone"; Harry: "School was absolutely boring") and perhaps start to misbehave (Wayne, who was disruptive as "I had no challenges") or be feared to be liable to start behaving badly (as was said of Tracy: "She's gonna be bored and she's gonna rebel soon"). On the teacher's part there could be a fear of how this might affect the other children:

> That was the same year they had a times table tournament and I stayed at the top of the tree so long that they actually had to stop it, because it was bad for everyone else's self-esteem apparently.

(Helene)

Or the teacher might display obliviousness as to how drawing attention to the gifted child's capability might place the child in an awkward position in relation to her peers, even bordering on humiliation:

> With spelling tests ... the teacher would say at the end "Okay, [Tracy], all those words now, you're going to tell the whole class what they all mean."
>
> *(Tracy)*

Whether the recognition was formal or informal, positive or negative, a frequent consequence would be that the extremely intelligent individual who was already in some way naturally standing out from others, would in some way be specifically set apart from others. The way of being set apart might be subtle, such as the way in which the child is referred to, or the way in which he or she notices an adult's reaction of being surprised or impressed. Or it might be very obvious, such as interviewee Helene who skipped two years of school or Gill who was put through her GCSE exams three years earlier than her peers.

Recognising something about yourself: effort and speed

So far we have focused on the environment's recognition of the high-IQ person's attributes, but something else that interviewees talked about is a recognition they came to on their part that they were different from others around them. The way they noticed this could be incremental, organic:

> There's no single point of time when I thought that this thing [high IQ] is manifesting itself, it's just that there would have been a time when I realised that something I was taking for granted was not so commonplace.
>
> *(Harry)*

Or there might have been a memorable moment for them when they came to this realisation:

> I expressed frustration that why aren't these people better at what they do? If they just tried they could just learn how to do it. And a friend of mine told me that no, actually, some people they may actually be trying right now. So I guess that's when I realised that, oh, okay, so maybe it is easier for me to learn similar things.
>
> *(Erik)*

Several interviewees spoke of the difficulty for them in working out what this difference meant for them and their relations with others:

> It's one of the great difficulties actually in interacting with other people, because you assume subconsciously that everyone else thinks the same way you do, everyone else functions the same way you do. And I don't think of myself on a day-to-day basis as a particularly ... well, as an extraordinarily unique human being.
>
> *(Helene)*

> It's the same obstacles but worse because you haven't been in someone else's head so you don't know that your head works much better, and even if along the way people tell you, "Oh you're quite smart", you don't put that into context because you have no context.
>
> *(Ana)*

> I do think being gifted, to be completely non-gifted or a low IQ in one way, it's the same disability because you then can't understand the norm.
>
> *(Mei)*

What my data showed was that a main differential that was repeatedly noticed between the extremely intelligent individual and others was within the dimensions of effort and speed. Over and over again I heard accounts of how interviewees had required much less effort than those around them in order to achieve the same result or better, and because it required less effort from them they would get to a result faster than others did.

> ... when I was at school, at primary school, I never carried my books back home. I never did homework because for me it was so easy at school, just in a break, like five minutes, I would do the homework very quickly.
>
> *(Don)*

> I remember ... especially on the math side, being able to finish it and grasp the concepts quicker than my peers.
>
> *(Sean)*

Adjectives to do with speed were regularly applied to their descriptions of their functioning:

> ... it frustrates the heck out of me to work in a team sometimes 'cos people are too slow. You just want people to get there quicker and they don't.
>
> *(Tracy)*

There were descriptions of their speed of verbal communication: "I talk fast" (Jane), or Ana:

> ... the best experience I ever had with a guy was he was as fast as me at understanding what I was about to say. We never had to finish sentences, we had the most condensed conversation ever possible because we were speaking at double speed half the time.

Descriptions of things being experienced as easy or "coming naturally" to them without effort were also frequent, for example: "I never bothered to learn anything, I just got it" (Mei); "Maths came very easy to me" (Wayne); "[IT] just comes naturally. It's not actually a lot of effort" (Hans); "I don't have to work for a lot of it. I have colleagues who sit for hours on end learning scores. I sing it twice and it's in here *[taps her head]*" (Helene). Two interviewees described having missed a lot of school – Paula through illness and Bonnie through truanting – and yet still having done well at their exams.

When an extremely intelligent individual comes to realise that he or she is different from others, what effect does this have? How does it make him or her feel? Don said:

> I feel sorry sometimes, because I, you know ... I see people working harder than me, but ... And they are not so lucky.

A few other interviewees also referred to themselves as lucky (e.g. Harry), and some expressed feeling sorry for others, expressing that "sometimes I think it's unfair" (Helene). Don added:

> It's something that I don't feel guilty [about] because it's not my fault, I never feel guilty but I would like it to be more fair.

Asserting "it's not my fault" involves a denial, and in this case it is a denial not of something that someone else has suggested to Don, but something that is in his own mind: he is the one who is introducing the concept of fault, through denying it. It appears therefore that the possibility that "it is my fault" is what has been felt first, however irrationally, prior to the discomfort of that possibility being defended against with a denial, wanting to be absolved of having any responsibility for the unfairness. Another example is Tracy speaking of her team at work being "slimmed down":

> ... so there's competition for places and it's clear that the management want me to stay, and it'll be at the expense of somebody else. I can't help that, they just know that I do a good job.

Saying "I can't help that" seems to suggest that she does feel bad that keeping her job will mean somebody else losing theirs, but that she is comforting or reassuring herself of no wrongdoing or culpability on her part. Mei spoke of specifically feeling guilty because her brother didn't do as well as she did and "my parents used me to compare me with him and it's completely unfair". She said that maybe it would have been better for him if she hadn't done so well. She went on to say that she feels *less* guilty about her achievements if she knows she's gifted, because "I couldn't help it, I'm just born that way". If she'd put in a lot of effort, then "it's like me trying to push everybody away from me". She said that she would feel guilty if it was her own will to "really leave everyone behind and just focus to get to where I am". However, by just doing her personal best at the tasks she is confronted with, "it's not something I plan to be ahead of everyone": "in that sense, it's almost like I'm helpless. To me gifted could be seen as a disability … we're just wired that way".

The recognition of high ability clearly brings about a grappling with how this affects others and how that in turn bears upon the extremely intelligent person's own conscience, with he or she having to do some internal work in order to arrive at feeling vindicated of blame for the unfairness of the observed differences in individual ability.

Being set apart versus belonging

We have seen above how the extremely intelligent individual who was already in some way naturally standing out from others, typically along the dimensions of effort and speed, would often then also – by the way that others would recognise and react to the differences involved – come to be specifically set apart from others. This could include the way in which their ability was pointed out by others or the way they were separated from others in groupings based on attainment.

Chapter 3 emphasised how crucial belonging in a group is for human beings, with the evolutionary rationale of gaining a group's assistance with protection and securing resources. Ingram & Morris (2007) explain that it is human nature to look for similarities in others and to identify with others, who one then groups together with. They term this "homophily" and place it at the core of socialisation. This relates to the work of Self Psychology pioneer Heinz Kohut who wrote about the developmental importance of what he called the "twinship transference" (1971), which essentially is the experience of alikeness that a person feels with another – feeling that you have shared characteristics between you. Experiencing alikeness, or twinship, with others, is what produces a sense of belonging with those others.

Given that the extremely intelligent child's particular biology and associated character traits and behaviours make him or her in certain aspects of experience and functioning dissimilar from at least 98% of the population, such a child might in their early influential environments encounter few, or zero, others who understand this and/or relate to this and/or themselves have similar experience and functioning. Legendary founder of Apple, Steve Jobs, was adopted as a baby, and as he was growing up he started to experience his significant dissimilarity from his adoptive parents in terms of intellectual functioning, making

82 Predicaments

him feel increasingly alienated from them (Isaacson 2011). Both the internal feeling of being different from others, and having the external environment treat you as different, can lead extremely intelligent individuals to feel that they don't fit in, they don't belong. As interviewee Gill said, "I often feel definitely the outsider in a group". Several other interviewees also used the term "outsider" for describing their experience. Wayne described a situation of not fitting in as follows:

> … at school there's two groups of people. You've got the first group … which is very well behaved and very academically minded, and you've got the group of rougher people who mess around and aren't really interested at school. So I was in the position where I had kudos with the academic ones because I was getting better test results than they were, but I used to hang around with the rougher lot … So in the end I worked out that I wasn't popular with either group because I didn't fit in the social circles of the better off and more academically minded children and I wanted to be [with] the rougher kids and muck around, play football, be naughty. But they always knew that I was clever as well so I wasn't really one of them either. So I was neither here nor there at school but I was good at passing exams.

The above excerpt introduces the socioeconomic aspect, where doing well academically is associated with being wealthier – "the better off *and* more academically minded" (my emphasis). This link was evident in other interviews also. For example Paula:

> … there were two girls who took an instant dislike to me and I think it was because I sounded slightly more posh than they did … they might've said something about being stuck up and clever.

Posh, stuck up, *and* clever. And there were interviewees who described distressing experiences of not fitting in not because of intellectual differences, but because their intellectual capacity had brought them into an environment with others of that capacity who were well-initiated into a socioeconomic culture and lifestyle that they were completely unfamiliar with.

> *[Talking about attending admissions interviews at a very prestigious university.]* We were sort of touted around parties and literally a sherry party. And we were all Mr and Miss surnames and it's just like off the scale of discomfort for me … I mean I was pained by this. Talking about sort of the shame, … I remember going down one morning and going into the wrong room for breakfast and literally sort of not quite twigging that everybody around me was some venerable old don. And then somebody came over and was, probably very kindly, but a little bit, "What are you

doing in here young man?" And I was just ... you know, I would have just eaten myself alive with embarrassment.

(John)

... it was just a total culture shock for me when I went to uni ... I couldn't relate to anybody, because I hadn't had any of the same experiences as them ... And I think my brain just shut down a little bit and it just went ... oh, I just can't deal with this. Yeah, I mean I lost two stone in about two months ... Just absolutely miserable and I just couldn't handle it ... If I hadn't had the issues at primary school, then it might not have, you know ... I hung around with people who were also very intelligent, also slightly socially awkward, you know like, because we got on with each other ... I hadn't fitted in for so long, to fit in with these people felt amazing. And then I got to uni and all of a sudden I didn't fit in with anybody again.

(Tess)

Both of these examples are about making a transition to a new environment, from school to university, where the interviewee came into contact with a different element of society for the first time, and one that is much more readily associated with intellectual achievement. Freeman (2010) also details a case where a gifted adolescent's abilities won her a place academically at a university which, on starting there, she could not adapt to socioculturally, causing her to drop out.

In what Tess says above, she makes it clear how important a feeling of fitting in or belonging was: after she had finally attained this at school, when it was then lost on starting university the effect on her was severe – losing two stone in weight, being "absolutely miserable", "brain just shut down", "just couldn't handle it". A feeling of not fitting in, not belonging with a group, is painful and anxiety-provoking, linked with the primitive fear of threat to survival that being rejected or abandoned could constitute and at the start of life did constitute.

Most of my interviewees mentioned ways of trying to find belonging. As Tess mentioned above, she had found a way of belonging with others who, like her, were "intelligent, also slightly socially awkward". She also said of this group "we got on with each other, but nobody else got on with us kind of thing". So here, those who do not feel they fit in form a group together so as to belong with each other. Tracy mentioned this also:

I remember teaming up with the unpopular kids, the girl who was ginger and everyone took the mick out of her because she was ginger, or this girl whose dad had died of a brain tumour, and everybody took the mick out of her. This is what children are like, they're horrible, but we banded together a little bit, an unpopular clique really to work against the popular kids.

Many interviewees spoke of longing for, or specifically seeking to be with, "like-minded" others, and the pure delight of feeling fully accepted and understood by others with whom a sense of belonging is felt. Tracy said of her partner:

> ... she's not threatened by it [high IQ], she loves it. She accepts it, she revels in it, she wants to learn from me, she wants to encourage me to ... she sits there, she does it all the time, she says, "Tell me about something, tell me about anything, explain something to me". If we're in the car or something, she'll say, "Tell me about Russia in the 19th century", or something and it's really lovely ...

The joy of this in a professional rather than personal context was described by interviewees who had experienced their abilities being fully engaged with together with others in the workplace with mutual appreciation and outcomes of effective joint enterprise. For example, Mei described her experience of belonging professionally with others similar to herself:

> So whenever I tell people that I've been with this company for 23 years, they all look a bit surprised but my view is ... that you don't get bored and you just always get stretched and also as I'm working with just clever people within the company, it's very stimulating and inspiring as well. I feel very comfortable with and enjoy their company as well, and we challenge each other in all sorts of ways.

The importance of belonging with a group for safety is shown for example by Paula. She talked about having had a group of friends – "... there's the four of us who were the strongest friends and we would've been the quite ... er ... geeky, swotty group I suppose" – who were split up when she started senior school and at that point, when she'd lost her group, was when she began to be bullied.

Another aspect of the attempt to safeguard a belonging with the group can manifest in the way that parents react to the recognition of extreme intelligence in their child.

> My teacher was trying to get my parents involved but because my parents were so working class ... to the point that on the back of the IQ test and my teacher's intervention, I was offered a place at a grammar school, a very prestigious grammar school in the area that I grew up, and my parents wouldn't let me go because they said, "You'll think badly of us".
>
> *(Tracy)*

In this example there is again the association between doing well academically and social class, and in this case a fear that a child will get separated from the family group if she is afforded opportunities for developing herself that have been foreign to her parents. Sadly, it was their holding back of her in an attempt to hold on to her that ultimately drove her away: she had "a massive row with my dad", moved out of home at age 17, and (for a period) "dropped out".

> I suppose I was quite resentful really of my parents because they didn't understand me remotely. They'd really stopped me from flowering if you like, and I knew that. I knew that when I was 11.

From my research it is apparent that the likelihood of intellectually gifted individuals coming into contact with similar and/or sympathetic others rises with the increased selectivity of the environment, and that the propensity for negative reaction is inversely proportionate to the number of similar and/or sympathetic others in the gifted individual's environment. This was evidenced with interviewees who experienced, for example, moving from a non-selective/mixed ability school to a selective one (e.g. Hans and Gill, presented in the previous chapter), and who found that the trouble with fitting in and being bullied ceased in the new environment.

Problems surrounding differentials in effort

It has been shown above that a main dimension that sets extremely intelligent individuals apart from others is the ratio of effort to achievement. As Gagné (2013:194) puts it, "ease and speed" in learning and acquiring expertise "are the trademarks of giftedness". In general our educational and occupational systems are set up in accordance with certain assumptions about what amount of effort is required for particular levels of achievement and at what stage therefore such achievement is expected to be reached. Where extremely intelligent individuals are concerned such assumptions and expectations are completely inaccurate. An example is provided by one of the largest prospective longitudinal studies on gifted children undertaken – the SMPY (the Study of Mathematically Precocious Youth) – which commenced in 1971 by Professor Julian Stanley of Johns Hopkins University. Participants were selected on the basis of having achieved extremely high SAT math scores at ages 11–13 (SAT tests are usually taken at age 16–17). Hunt (2011:346) reports that "The SMPY students could assimilate a year's high school course work in about three weeks of intensive study". It is also this dimension of differentials in effort and speed that causes in others the most awe, and in the gifted individual, the most bewilderment, frustration, and adjustment difficulty.

> I can see that I can get there but he couldn't. I couldn't explain why he couldn't get there very quickly and I think this is my problem as well, I probably arrived at an answer very quickly even with normal maths problems, but I'm very bad at explaining to people how I got there,

I just got there, I don't need all these steps and I can't explain how these steps go.

(Mei)

[Speaking of her extremely intelligent mother.] She would describe herself as a mad scientist and her style of thinking is very A, B, Z. She doesn't have to go through C, D, E, F, G, which is something I seem to have inherited, so's my sister. But that causes problems with colleagues who don't understand how you're getting the result or reaching the conclusion that you've reached quite logically to you, but it causes friction in a workplace.

(Helene)

It is understandably inconvenient for systems to encounter individuals who do not suit the system. In general, however, educational systems are far readier to make adaptations to cater for individuals who are lagging behind the expected level of achievement than they are to make adaptations for those who are speeding ahead. In family systems also, speeding ahead can be reacted to with disapproval and discouragement, such as interviewee Tracy's experience while growing up of being told repeatedly that "I should not get ahead of myself".

The phrase "don't get ahead of yourself" is intriguing, because it appears that it could well mean that it is *others*, rather than yourself, that you are being warned not to get ahead of. Or others' ideas of where you are or should be, of what your correct place is. The saying "getting ahead of yourself" is similar to that of "being out of order" or "out of line". One of the ways that this manifests in families, is in relation to birth order, which can impose a kind of hierarchy that there is an implicit rule to respect: Tracy told how she was three years younger than her sister but "a lot cleverer" and was shooting ahead of her, which caused difficulty as it contravened the naturally expected order of things. John used the phrase "out of line" in describing his behaviour that elicited his father's violent attempts to stop his precocious questioning. Harry talked about a traditional hierarchically organised profession where you had to "join at the back of the queue" and could not "jump out of the queue" – you could not be promoted over someone who was chronologically older than you were. In these situations, respect for the existing order is being demanded rather than a person's ability and contribution being welcomed or assessed on their own merits regardless of whether he or she is a child, a younger sibling, or a more junior employee.

When "speeding ahead" is resisted and deterred, this shows that the individual difference that underlies the capacity to speed ahead is an individual difference that is regarded as something that it is alright to neglect. It is assumed that the person concerned should just put up with it, that if it is ignored it will hopefully go away or be fine. It is not regarded as something that, if not adequately catered for, can lead to serious personal and social problems. Favier-Townsend

(2014) has documented some of the long-term problems this causes, and how "intellectual neglect" in childhood can lead to underachievement that is linked with poor mental health in adulthood. She argued that giftedness should be recognised as a SEN (Special Educational Need).

When gifted individuals are in an environment where very little effort is needed from them to stay abreast of the level of achievement that is expected of them and being demonstrated by their peers, they do not acquire the habit of disciplined, persistent effort that is necessary to accomplish anything of real importance (Hollingworth 1942; Towers 1987; Grobman 2006). Developing lazy habits means that if they later find themselves facing challenges that they are unable to meet with little effort, they either avoid the challenge, or fail at it. The former establishes a pattern of underachievement, while the latter can be experienced as devastating because the praise they have received for their prior effortless achievement builds an identity as an achiever that they can become dependent on for their self-esteem and which is then threatened.

Mueller & Dweck (1998) showed that the way a person's achievement is reacted to shapes his or her subsequent attitude and behaviour. When children are praised for their intelligence, it can change their goals from task engagement, enjoyment, and the gaining of learning, to the goal of trying to keep looking smart to others. They can also lose motivation, shifting from doing things for internal reasons to doing things for external rewards. Subsequent performance suffers. They feel pressured to produce future good performance, and, as their self-worth becomes contingent on doing well, they react maladaptively to achievement setbacks, manifesting negative affect, negative self-cognitions, and avoidance of further challenges rather than displaying resilience and persistence. In spite of all of these difficult outcomes associated with praising a child for his or her intelligence, Mueller & Dweck (1998) also showed that it is highly common for people to praise ability (rather than effort).

In terms of self-concept, confidence is built by experiencing effort leading to achievement (Colangelo et al. 1993), so if achievement is attained without effort it is not valued and does not build a sense of internal control and confidence. If others insist on lauding such achievement, those others are perceived as ignorant, out of touch, because they do not understand how meaningless the event has been for the extremely intelligent person. Grobman (2006:207) reports a gifted patient of his saying that her accomplishments had been "as easy as breathing", and "should I feel proud of breathing?" That is also why such persons can feel they are a fake or a fraud, termed "imposter syndrome" (Clance & Imes 1978), because they experience that they are being praised for something that for them has not constituted what they would regard as an achievement, and which they have not internalised as an achievement, because it did not involve effort for them. Also, not experiencing competition from others denies high-IQ individuals the opportunity to build confidence by engaging in challenging competition with those who are a good match for them (Khan 2005).

From the classroom to the courtroom

A different way that a recognition of one's own ability can develop, is that the extremely intelligent individual becomes disdainful towards others because of experiencing them as being slow, incapable, having a futile focus or setting ridiculous restrictions, and develops cynicism about systems and disrespect for rules. This kind of attitude, coupled with the boredom that such an individual often feels within the routines of ordinary school or workplace systems, can cause him or her to rebel (as interviewee Tracy's teachers had feared) or to start to "misbehave" as Wayne did, or to truant as Bonnie did. Harry described:

> The subjects that I enjoyed I would read the entire textbook within the first couple of weeks. The subjects that I didn't like at all I would probably never read any of it ever, but that really meant that in class I would be with my friends pulling pranks or creating some kind of disturbance in class.

Not being understood by or suitably catered for and challenged by the teachers and school system can lead to acquiring "a contempt for authority that will carry over into adulthood, causing … lifelong problems" (Towers 1987:1). As a way to create for themselves the stimulation and challenges that are lacking from their environment, gifted children can turn to cheating, dishonesty, and manipulation, exercising their surplus ability and energy by seeking shortcuts, loopholes, and ways to buck the system (Maupin 2014). Often they are motivated purely by wanting to see if something is actually possible, and often they are clever enough to pull it off and remain undetected (Maupin 2014). Getting away with it can create a burgeoning sense of personal power. A client of mine described never having had a sense of "a lack of invincibility," and another enthused about how, together with a few "over-achieving" friends, "we were masters of the universe!" High achievement can lead to more of a sense of power, as well as to more actual power, success, influence, admiration, and even fame, which can engender even more of a sense of invincibility. And if satisfying (and legal) channels for high ability are not found, the cheating of childhood can translate in adulthood into criminal activity, often at high levels of sophistication, which can similarly go undetected. Although a strong correlation has been well-evidenced of criminal behaviour decreasing with increasing IQ (e.g. Beaver et al. 2013), what is less known is that it has also been shown that when reaching the very highest levels of IQ, the crime line suddenly rises (Schwartz et al. 2015). A study on genius-level IQ – scores of 150 and higher – found a higher prevalence of criminal activity in this group (centred on white-collar crime, property offences, and professional misconduct) (Oleson 2016). And in terms of detection, Boccioa et al. (2018) found that individuals with higher verbal IQ are more likely to avoid arrest for criminal behaviour.

Steven Spielberg's 2002 film *Catch Me If You Can* – spoiler alert – dramatises the true story of Frank Abagnale (played by Leonardo DiCaprio), one of the most daring and successful con artists in history. Tom Hanks plays the FBI agent Carl Hanratty who follows his trail. Abagnale achieved millions of dollars' worth of cheque fraud before the age of 21, and successfully posed as an airline pilot and a doctor. However, what Hanratty is most intrigued by when he finally does catch up with Abagnale, is how Abagnale, who had no university education, managed to secure the job he got as a lawyer, for which study of about seven years is required plus the passing of the notoriously difficult bar exam. Hanratty keeps asking him how he managed to cheat at the bar exam. Eventually Abagnale reveals that he did not cheat. In reality Abagnale forged himself a Harvard law degree transcript with which to register for the bar exam, and then passed the exam after studying for it for four months (Abagnale & Redding 1980). The condensing of about seven years of study into four months is an impressive feat of extreme intelligence.

A motivation for a very high-IQ person committing crime can be, as Abagnale described it – a seeking of "the thrill of the scam" (cited in Maupin 2014:242). Or they can do it simply because they realise they can, such as an accountant client of mine who was convicted of embezzlement and said the large corporation involved "had been asking for it" as their procedures were so slack. Here the attitude of disdain is apparent, where personal culpability is ignored in favour of the system being mocked and blamed, and the individual's breach of the responsibility that he or she was entrusted with is disregarded. This example also demonstrates greed as a factor, which is what was said to be a main motivation when another case of extremely intelligent crime came to prominence, in the form of Tom Hayes's dishonest manipulation of LIBOR (the London Interbank Offered Rate) – "the biggest banking crime in history" (Connett 2015b) – which had global impact and reaped profits of hundreds of millions of dollars. Hayes was said to have developed a "God syndrome" (Connett 2015a) in the way he exercised his intellectual prowess, prior to being sentenced to 14 years' imprisonment. As with Abagnale and Hayes – and my interviewee Bonnie who spent four years in jail – in many of these cases the daring and contravention of legal limits does eventually result in criminal justice. Boccioa et al.'s (2018) study showed that the law of probability meant that, with repeated offence, high-IQ offenders were apprehended almost at the same rate as low-IQ offenders who had committed a similar number of crimes. In Lin-Manuel Miranda's (2015) song "Non-stop" from the musical *Hamilton*, the attitudes and actions of the extremely intelligent Alexander Hamilton (one of the seven Founding Fathers of the United States) are being interrogated by the person who becomes his deadly adversary, Aaron Burr. Burr questions why Hamilton always assumes he is the "smartest in the room" and warns that this attitude may be his "doom". It is this kind of sequence of events that is being cautioned against in the numerous mythological tales of hubris leading to nemesis.

The dynamics of envy: a compassion barrier

We have seen how the individual differences of very high-IQ persons not being catered for can lead to destructiveness and loss and have impact at personal, societal, and even global levels. What, then, is the reason for such resistance to acknowledging, and catering compassionately for, the needs of extremely intelligent individuals? It appears, in essence, to be insecurity: witnessing someone "speeding ahead" triggers the visceral threat-detection reaction of fearing "being left behind". This is apparent in parents who try to turn away from and ignore or suppress their child's high IQ, and in teachers who react negatively to a pupil's precocity rather than positively embracing it and investing in it.

Whole cultures can act to deter such "speeding ahead", for example in Australia where the phenomenon is termed "cutting down tall poppies". Australian researcher Norman Feather (2012) has extensively studied this phenomenon. He has demonstrated that the perception of "deservingness" is a key variable in how people react to successes and failures in themselves and others (Feather et al. 2011). He found that successes were judged as being undeserved, and resented, if these were perceived as having been achieved with little effort (Feather & Sherman 2002). When a success was followed by a failure, misfortune, or fall from grace, this was greeted with more *Schadenfreude* (pleasure) in direct proportion to how undeserving the initial success was judged to have been (Feather & Sherman 2002). By virtue of the fact that an extremely intelligent individual requires far less effort in relation to achievement than does the average person, gifted/high-IQ individuals are particularly vulnerable to having others rejoice in their misfortune, which is the opposite of compassion.

Extremely intelligent individuals can find themselves in a no-win situation. If they allow the extent of their effortless achievement to be apparent to others, they court resentment. However, if others interpret their achievement as surely having required a lot of effort, the gifted individual can be perceived as someone who has "just kept studying all the time and had no social life" (as interviewee Max said people had falsely assumed of him), or who is aggressively competitive and has specifically tried to "leave others behind" (rather than, "I was just born that way, it's not my fault", as Mei said). Mei described that she felt better about herself if she knew she had not specifically put effort in to excel beyond others, to "leave others behind", but noticed (echoing Feather's findings) that others seemed to feel better about her and could be more accepting of her achievement if her achievement appeared to them to have cost her some significant effort, rather than that it came easily to her. Either way, it is difficult for extremely intelligent individuals to find in others an understanding of, and empathy with, the reality of their experience.

Feather (1989) found that people who favoured the fall of tall poppies, and reported more *Schadenfreude*, tended to be lower in self-esteem, power, and achievement, to set a higher value on equality, and to be more left wing. It is clear from this that for gifted individuals to feel able to freely express themselves, and to be acknowledged and given encouragement and support, they need to be in an environment with others who understand their unique predicament around effort and achievement, or who are themselves similar and/or who are themselves robust in self-esteem, power, and achievement.

Schadenfreude is, of course, a version of envy: envy involves coveting what advantage someone else seems to have (related to which is jealousy, which is feeling envious resentment towards someone for their perceived advantage). The hallmark of envy is a reaction that tries to spoil what someone has. Spoiling can involve taking pleasure in someone's misfortune, or marring their joy by criticising or withholding interest in something they are enthusiastic about, or withholding commendation for their efforts or achievements. Envious behaviours can include obstruction and even open hostility, such as colleagues protecting their own territory by blocking someone, excluding them, or putting them down to try to stop that person looking good. As interviewee Avi said: "Envy means they are going to start building walls and barriers".

Wishing to spoil things for someone arises out of wishing to destroy the advantage that person is perceived to have. And the main reason for wishing to destroy what is perceived as another person's advantage, is that it is seen as posing a threat to oneself. Seeing what is capable or admirable in a person could make you feel, in relation to that person, less good about yourself, and can make you fear that that person will – because of what's capable or admirable in them – deprive you of something that matters to you (e.g. your perceived attractiveness to or worth to others, your status, or a job or promotion). Interviewee Helene reported her mother having explained this to her as follows:

> You have to understand that they feel less, because … you seem to be more … They feel threatened by that.

However, even when there is no actual threat, these dynamics of envy can become a psychological habit that is triggered automatically when perceiving something good that someone else has (which can even be irrespective of whether you have something equivalent yourself). What is clear is that one of the barriers that this can erect is a compassion barrier: it is generally much easier to feel compassionate towards someone who is in some way worse off than oneself, rather than towards someone who is in some way better off than oneself. A psychotherapist colleague described to me how she gave a presentation in which she discussed two cases she had worked with. At the end of the presentation, a member of the audience said, with some horror or disapproval, "You show as much compassion for the fine art collecting banking lawyer as you do for the patient who has been abused from the cradle". As though that was wrong. My colleague said she thought this marvellously showed something of the difficulty people can have with those whom they see as being more privileged than themselves.

It is no wonder that gifted individuals can become adept at hiding their abilities and achievements to protect themselves from this form of hostility from others that they are uniquely vulnerable to. Thirteen out of my first 16 interviewees spoke about doing this in one way or another. This could involve instances of hiding their full abilities, achievements, or affiliations in order to ward off interpersonal difficulty that was being experienced or being anticipated. For example, several mentioned that they never disclose that they are members of Mensa. Hiding something specific in a particular context can be a sensible decision, and this is different from a more overall hiding of self. For example, interviewee Harry spoke about a permanent hiding of himself, in all situations: he avoided social contact because of the effort of having to "put on my mask", and described fearing that others "might discover who I am". In such cases the person has made a change to themselves that might entail never fully expressing themselves spontaneously, and they may not even be aware of how extreme this hiding of self has become.

Summary

This chapter has charted how the manifestations of extreme intelligence – particularly in terms of differentials between high-IQ/gifted individuals and others in effort and speed – come to be recognised by self and others, and what sorts of intrapersonal and interpersonal reactions this can trigger. Such reactions can range from a sense of guilt at the unfairness of the individual differences involved, and high-IQ underachievement, through to hubris and high-IQ crime. Building on the core concepts from the previous chapter, this has been explored in relation to the themes of belonging and competing: high ability can help a person to compete successfully but can also make an extremely intelligent person feel like – and be treated as – an outsider. Typical attendant difficulties of envy and a breakdown in compassion and empathy have been explained, together with very high-IQ individuals' attempts to protect themselves against these difficulties by hiding their true abilities. Concepts drawn on to demonstrate the importance of belonging have included homophily (Ingram & Morris) and twinship transference (Kohut). The relevance of Feather's work on "cutting down tall poppies" and *Schadenfreude,* and Mueller & Dweck's on the effects of praise, has been considered. These themes have been evidenced throughout with a presentation and analysis of excerpts from my research interviews. In the next chapter we will look further into the kinds of predicaments that can arise interpersonally between extremely intelligent individuals and others as a result of the kinds of differences in functioning between them.

References

Abagnale, F. W. & Redding, S. (1980). *Catch Me If You Can*. Edinburgh: Mainstream Publishing Company.

Beaver, K. M., Schwartz, J. A., Nedelec, J. L., Connolly, E. J., Boutwell, B. B. & Barnes, J. C. (2013). Intelligence is associated with criminal justice processing: arrest through incarceration. *Intelligence*, 41, pp. 277–288.

Boccioa, C. M., Beavera, K. M. & Schwartzc, J. A. (2018). The role of verbal intelligence in becoming a successful criminal: results from a longitudinal sample. *Intelligence*, 66, pp. 24–31.

Clance, P. R. & Imes, S. A. (1978). The imposter phenomenon in high achieving women: dynamics and therapeutic intervention. *Psychotherapy: Theory, Research and Practice*, 15(3), pp. 241–247.

Colangelo, N., Kerr, B., Christensen, P. & Maxey, J. (1993). A comparison of gifted underachievers and gifted achievers. *Gifted Child Quarterly*, 37(4), pp. 15–160.

Connett, D. (2015a). Tom Hayes developed a "God syndrome", court hears in Libor trial. *Independent*. [online] Available at: www.independent.co.uk/news/business/news/libor-trial-trader-tom-hayes-developed-a-god-syndrome-court-hears-a6693171.html. [Accessed 13 March 2019].

Connett, D. (2015b). Libor scandal: discovering what lay behind Tom Hayes' decision to rig interest rates. *Independent*. [online] Available at: www.independent.co.uk/news/business/news/libor-scandal-discovering-what-lay-behind-tom-hayes-decision-to-rig-interest-rates-10436389.html. [Accessed 13 March 2019].

Eccles, J. S. (1999). The development of children ages 6 to 14. *The Future of Children*, 9(2), pp. 30–44.

Erikson, E. H. (1950). *Childhood and Society*. New York: W. W. Norton & Company.

Erikson, E. H. (1968). *Identity: Youth and Crisis*. New York: W. W. Norton & Company.

Favier-Townsend, A. (2014). *Perceived Causes and Long Term Effects of Delayed Academic Achievement in High IQ Adults*. Unpublished PhD thesis, University of Hertfordshire, UK.

Feather, N. (2012). Tall poppies, deservingness and schadenfreude. *The Psychologist*, 25(6), pp. 434–437.

Feather, N. T. (1989). Attitudes towards the high achiever: the fall of the tall poppy. *Australian Journal of Psychology*, 41, pp. 239–267.

Feather, N. T., McKee, I. R. & Bekker, N. (2011). Deservingness and emotions. *Motivation and Emotion*, 35, pp. 1–13.

Feather, N. T. & Sherman, R. (2002). Envy, resentment, schadenfreude, and sympathy. *Personality and Social Psychology Bulletin*, 28, pp. 953–961.

Freeman, J. (2010). *Gifted Lives: What Happens When Gifted Children Grow Up*. London: Routledge.

Freud, S. (1914). On narcissism: an introduction. In: J. Strachey (Ed.). *The Standard Edition of the Complete Psychological Works of Sigmund Freud Volume XIV*. Reprint 2001. London: Vintage, pp. 67–102.

Gagné, F. (2013). Yes, giftedness (aka "innate" talent) does exist! In: S. B. Kaufman (Ed.). *The Complexity of Greatness*. Oxford: Oxford University Press, pp. 191–221.

Garfinkel, H. (1956). Conditions of successful degradation ceremonies. *The American Journal of Sociology*, 61, pp. 420–424.

Grobman, J. (2006). Underachievement in exceptionally gifted adolescents and young adults: a psychiatrist's view. *The Journal of Gifted Secondary Education*, 17, pp. 199–209.

Hollingworth, L. S. (1942). *Children above 180 IQ: Their Origin and Development*. New York: World Books.

Hunt, E. (2011). *Human Intelligence*. New York: Cambridge University Press.

Ingram, P. & Morris, M. W. (2007). Do people mix at mixers? Structure, homophily, and the 'life of the party'. *Administrative Science Quarterly*, 52(4), pp. 558–585.

Isaacson, W. (2011). *Steve Jobs: The Exclusive Biography*. New York: Simon & Schuster.

Kaufman, S. B. (2008). *Is Every Child Gifted? Probably Not.* [online] Available at: www.psychologytoday.com/blog/beautiful-minds/200805/is-every-child-gifted-probably-not. [Accessed 12 September 2016].

Khan, M. (2005). *Gifted Achievers and Underachievers: An Appraisal.* India: Discovery Publishing House.

Kohut, H. (1971). *The Analysis of the Self.* Reprint 2009. Chicago, IL: University of Chicago Press.

Magee, J. C. & Galinsky, A. D. (2009). Social hierarchy: the self-reinforcing nature of power and status. *The Academy of Management Annals*, 2(1), pp. 351–398.

Maupin, K. (2014). *Cheating, Dishonesty and Manipulation: Why Bright Kids Do It.* Tucson, AZ: Great Potential Press.

Mueller, C. M. & Dweck, C. S. (1998). Praise for intelligence can undermine children's motivation and performance. *Journal of Personality and Social Psychology*, 75(1), pp. 33–52.

Oleson, J. C. (2016). *Criminal Genius: A Portrait of High-IQ Offenders.* Oakland, CA: University of California Press.

Ossorio, P. G. (2006). *The Behavior of Persons.* Ann Arbor, MI: Descriptive Psychology Press.

Roosevelt, T. (n.d.). *Quotes.* [online] Available at: https://en.wikiquote.org/wiki/Theodore_Roosevelt. [Accessed 12 September 2016].

Sapolsky, R. M. (2005). The influence of social hierarchy on primate health. *Science*, 308 (5722), pp. 648–652.

Schwartz, J. A., Savolainen, J., Aaltonen, M., Merikukka, M., Paananen, R. & Gissler, M. (2015). Intelligence and criminal behavior in a total birth cohort: an examination of functional form, dimensions of intelligence, and the nature of offending. *Intelligence*, 51, pp. 108–118.

Schwartz, W. (1979). Degradation, accreditation, and rites of passage. *Psychiatry*, 42, pp. 138–146.

Sharma, A. & Cockerill, H. (2014). *Mary Sheridan's from Birth to Five Years: Children's Developmental Progress.* (4th ed.). London: Routledge.

Sherman, G. D., Lee, J. J., Cuddy, A. J. C., Renshon, J., Oveis, C., Gross, J. J. & Lerner, J. S. (2012). Leadership is associated with lower levels of stress. *Proceedings of the National Academy of Sciences of the United States of America (PNAS)*, 109(44), pp. 17,903–17,907.

The Holy Bible, English Standard Version. (2012). London: HarperCollins Publishers.

Towers, G. M. (1987). The outsiders. *Gift of Fire*, 22. [online] Available at: www.cpsimoes.net/artigos/outsiders.html. [Accessed 5 February 2017].

Wilkinson, R. (2001). *Mind the Gap: Hierarchies, Health and Human Evolution.* London: Yale University Press.

Yermish, A. (2010). *Cheetahs on the Couch: Issues Affecting the Therapeutic Working Alliance with Clients Who are Cognitively Gifted.* Unpublished PhD thesis, Massachusetts School of Professional Psychology.

5
NAIVE CHILD, ARROGANT EMPEROR
Are the intellectually adept, socially inept?

> **Reflective Prompt 5:** If you were asked whether you think that highly intelligent people typically experience social problems, would you say yes or no? On what information or experience is your answer based? Do you know, or know of, someone who you think of as being extremely intelligent, who appears to have difficult relationships? What do you see as causing this person's trouble with others: for example, can you identify something that he or she keeps doing, or keeps failing to do, that creates problems?

British psychologist and specialist in gifted children, Professor Joan Freeman, mentions the stereotype that gifted individuals are strange, referring to the "popular image" (2010:7) of the gifted child as lonely, with painful problems. American psychiatrist and psychotherapist Dr Jerald Grobman, who specialises in consulting with gifted individuals, writes that none of his patients liked being called gifted – they thought it connoted being odd, troubled, or just plain different, and that none liked feeling different from their friends (Grobman 2009). Why has such a negative stereotype formed of extremely intelligent individuals? What basis – if any – is there for this in fact?

This chapter explores the stereotype of the extremely intelligent person as eccentric or socially dysfunctional. It starts with examples of depictions of this in characters in novels, history, and the media. Manifestations of this are then analysed in the academic literature and in excerpts from my research interviews where a theme was identified of very high IQ being paired with interpersonal difficulty.

The stereotype of the extremely intelligent person as socially inept

This stereotype comes in various versions, ranging from a person who is highly intellectually capable (Gf) and knowledgeable (Gc) being somewhat benignly incompetent at day-to-day practicalities, to such a person being substantially offensive. Beginning with the benign, we have the "absent-minded professor" stereotype, as depicted in this excerpt from a children's novel:

> He was a wizard – a small man with thin arms and legs and an absolutely enormous head almost entirely filled with brains ... and there was nothing he hadn't learnt ... [H]e had seven university degrees ... But he didn't have any degrees in Everyday Life.
>
> *(Ibbotson 2010:12)*

This fictional character is endowed with the empirically evidenced correlation between brain size and intellect. Another fictional character famous for her intelligence is Harry Potter's friend Hermione Granger (although they do not start as friends). The very first phrase with which she is introduced to us when she makes her entrance in the first of the seven novels, is "she had a bossy sort of voice" (Rowling 1997:79). And her very first social interaction with the other characters involves her openly speaking her mind and being critical towards them ("Are you sure that's a real spell? ... Well, it's not very good, is it?"), followed by her displaying her own proficiency ("I've tried a few simple spells just for practise and it's all worked for me") (Rowling 1997:79). Hot on the heels of this she demonstrates her love of learning, achievement orientation, and speed of functioning: she says, "I've learnt all our set books off by heart, of course, I just hope it will be enough", and it is described that "she said all of this very fast" (Rowling 1997:79). The first description of how other characters first react to her – a "stunned face" (Rowling 1997:79) – shows that she has managed to instantaneously breach their ordinary expectations and implicit social conventions. In other words, she stands out as being very different from them. And what this triggers is prompt rejection: the first thing any of the other characters says of her is "Whatever house I'm in, I hope she's not in it" (Rowling 1997:80).

The contradicting of ordinary social expectations is a hallmark feature of this stereotype. Alan Turing, pre-eminent mathematician whose code-breaking transformed the Second World War and who designed the first digital computer, has been described as socially having had "off-hand manners", "long silences", "a strange way of not meeting the eye", and as being "brusque" and "one who never fitted in anywhere quite successfully" (Irvine 2012:xix–xxi). Probably the most astoundingly high-achieving contemporary personality whose name is commonly recognised and encountered in the media, is SpaceX and Tesla CEO Elon Musk. His turbulent personal life includes being twice divorced. It is described that he "can come off as shy and borderline awkward" (Vance 2015:8) and that while growing up "those around him judged that he was either rude or really weird," which "didn't endear him to his peers" (Vance 2015:32).

An associated regular feature apparent in this, is that of the consequences in social rejection. Both Turing and Musk were badly bullied at school. Iconoclastic philosopher Arthur Schopenhauer was even ultimately rejected by his own mother, Johanna Schopenhauer. In one of her letters to him, she wrote:

> You irritate me no end and you are extremely difficult to deal with. Your extreme intelligence casts a dark cloud over your good characteristics – so nobody can benefit from them ... you criticize everything and everyone, except yourself ... so it is not surprising that you become alienated from the people close to you. Nobody enjoys being corrected or exposed.
> *(cited in Nauta & Ronner 2013)*

Remembering (from Chapter 3) that social rejection activates the same part of the brain that is activated by physical pain, the examples of these individuals not securing acceptance or belonging can immediately arouse our compassion. However, it becomes more complex when taking into consideration the pain that these individuals themselves inflict on others. For example, Musk "sets unrealistic goals, verbally abuses employees, and works them to the bone" (Vance 2015:17). These are the exact same severe behaviours ascribed to Steve Jobs (Isaacson 2011). This is where benign social eccentricity shades into substantial interpersonal difficulty. How prevalent is this connecting of interpersonal difficulty with extreme intelligence?

The academic literature: asserting versus denying interpersonal difficulties

In the literature and research on giftedness – the vast majority of which pertains to children, not adults – there are ubiquitous references to interpersonal problems. Some of these references involve assertions of interpersonal problems, for example Webb et al. (2016) who maintain that the characteristics of giftedness strongly influence relationships and can lead to significant problems and a clinically significant impairment in functioning (also Neihart et al. 2002). Guenole et al. (2015) assert that it is common for intellectually gifted children to be referred to paediatric or child neuropsychiatry clinics for socio-emotional problems. Other references involve denials that there are such problems, such as Freeman (2013), and Jones's (2013) meta-analysis of studies on children. There is empirical support for both positions (Neihart 1999; Lopez & Sotillo 2009), i.e. that gifted individuals function well socially and that they do not function well socially. I have not found any studies that differentiate between interpersonal relating in a general social situation as opposed to more intimate one-to-one interpersonal relating. What is clear, however, is that whether interpersonal difficulty is being asserted or denied, there is a widespread presence of this issue being considered, researched, and debated in relation to very high-IQ individuals.

There are many reasons for the conflicting results. One difference might relate to the age at which participants are evaluated. Peyre et al. (2016) did not find in preschool children more behavioural, emotional, and social problems in those with high IQ as compared with those with normal IQ. However, a longitudinal study that assessed 1,326 high-IQ individuals in adolescence and again 30 years later, found that high-IQ individuals had better adjustment than those with average IQ during adolescence but "moderately worse" adjustment in midlife (with lower global life satisfaction and satisfaction with friend relations) (Zettergren 2014). Another reason for different results relates to the source of the sample. Studies that obtain a gifted sample by recruiting from gifted educational programmes or groups of proven high achievers (e.g. American Presidential Scholars – see Kaufmann & Matthews 2012), are accessing participants who have already been selected for being able to function successfully rather than ones who might be experiencing difficulties that could impede their achievement. Neihart (1999) found three factors that influence psychological outcomes across different age groups: the type of giftedness, the educational fit, and personal characteristics. A further difference was confirmed in a study by Guenole et al. (2015), which found that children with significant discrepancies between scores on the verbal versus performance assessments on Wechsler's intelligence profile are more emotionally and behaviourally impaired than high-IQ children who have a more even profile.

Another reason for different results lies in the kind of research methodology employed. For example, quantitative questionnaires can be susceptible to a social desirability skewing effect (De Vellis 2012), with research participants answering according to how they would like to present themselves publicly rather than according to what their more private experience actually is. By contrast, one-to-one confidential qualitative research interviews can provide participants with an experience of "recognition and containment" (Hollway & Jefferson 2013:45–47) that promotes more candour in their responses. In my own mixed methods research I found that the same individuals who did not declare any mental health difficulties on their questionnaires, in interview opened up and revealed struggles of this kind (Falck 2013).

The earliest studies on giftedness, by Terman (1925) and Hollingworth (1942), made associations between higher IQ and social maladjustment. The essence of this is that an extremely intelligent person has cognitive functioning that is so different from that of the majority of people – at least two standard deviations away from the norm on the Bell Curve (see Introduction) – that they are not understood by, and cannot understand, the majority of others, and this is what produces difficulty in social interaction.

> A lesson which many gifted persons never learn as long as they live is that human beings in general are inherently very different from themselves in

thought, in action, in general intention, and in interests ... This is one of the most painful and difficult lessons that each gifted child must learn, if personal development is to proceed successfully... Failure to learn how to tolerate in a reasonable fashion the foolishness of others leads to bitterness, disillusionment, and misanthropy.

(Hollingworth 1942:259)

A much more recent echo of this is found in Detterman's (2014) description of how high ability students are often shocked when they realise that others do not function the same way they do.

There can be very different experiences associated with different bands of high IQ (Ruf 2009), and the higher the IQ, the more the problems. Hollingworth (1942) asserted that those in the high IQ range of 130–150 experience better adjustment than those with IQ above 150. To emphasise how rare this score is, those with IQs of 150 and above occur about 5–7 times out of 10,000 persons (Powell & Haden 1984). We saw in the previous chapter how very much faster a gifted child masters a school curriculum in comparison with his or her age peers. But as most schools are arranged in age groups, such a child will often not have intellectual equals in the peer group. Hollingworth (1942:262) defined the nature of the interpersonal problems involved as centring on "suffering fools" and becoming isolated:

> These superior children are not unfriendly or ungregarious by nature. Typically they strive to play with others but their efforts are defeated by the difficulties of the case ... Other children do not share their interests, their vocabulary, or their desire to organize activities ... As a result, forms of solitary play develop, and these, becoming fixed as habits, may explain the fact that many highly intellectual adults are shy, ungregarious, and unmindful of human relationships, or even misanthropic and uncomfortable in ordinary social intercourse.

As Towers (1987b:1–2) puts it,

> If he manages to resist forming attitudes of rebellion and cynicism, he may find companionship in learned societies and the like when he reaches adulthood. But even so, he frequently never overcomes the habits of solitude, shyness, and self-depreciation that were forged for him in childhood.

Webb et al. (2016:274) cite educational psychologist and prominent intelligence researcher Arthur Jensen as having stated in a personal communication that there is a "zone of tolerance" of about 20 IQ points. Towers maintains that a difference of 30 IQ points between individuals creates a communication barrier, and a child who is different by that much from the majority of, or all of, those around him or her, has a childhood "not unlike that of the deaf" child (1987a:1).

A Dutch study conducted on gifted adults rather than children examined the personality characteristics of 196 Mensa members (Dijkstra et al. 2012). Results showed that these individuals of 98th percentile or higher IQ, compared with a general community sample, showed lower levels of conscientiousness, agreeableness, extraversion, and emotional intelligence. In addition, among the gifted adults conscientiousness was positively related to well-being, whereas in the comparison group extraversion was positively related to well-being (Dijkstra et al. 2012). My own research showed that a sample of 229 British Mensa members had an atypical profile of attachment styles, with a much higher percentage of insecure – predominantly avoidant – attachment than in general populations (Falck 2013), which is associated with greater interpersonal difficulty. Both of these latter two studies suggest lower levels of social engagement in gifted adults.

For me the issue is not to seek an ultimate ruling on whether extremely intelligent individuals tend to have trouble with interpersonal relating or not, it is about finding out, where there is difficulty, how this arises, what the nature of it is, and what can be done about it. My interest is also in exploring, where there is not such difficulty, what makes the difference between those who do and those who do not (or do not any longer) experience such difficulty. So, how does interpersonal difficulty in very high-IQ individuals arise?

Causes: how difficulty arises

Jacobsen (1999b) sees relationship problems in very high-IQ individuals as expressions of problems with what she designates as the three hallmarks of giftedness: complexity, intensity, and drive. She writes about how such individuals shock others with their intensity, exhaust them with their complexity, and overwhelm them with their drive. There is support from other authors for each of these (Lovecky 1986; Streznewski 1999; Daniels & Piechowski 2009; Fonseca 2016; Webb et al. 2016; Heylighen, n.d.a; n.d.b). Drive can be expressed through high energy and perfectionism, and complexity means that highly intelligent individuals see things from more angles, and in more depth, than others do or want to, which can cause others confusion. Such complexity can delay decisions and cause frustration for all concerned. The way that other hallmark characteristics of giftedness (introduced in Chapter 3) are documented to cause interpersonal difficulty are as follows:

> *Asynchrony:* Being cognitively – but not emotionally – much more advanced than others of their age can make gifted individuals stand out from others, confuse others' expectations, and be difficult to manage particularly in groups that are organised according to age (Webb et al. 2016). This can be exacerbated if dual or multiple exceptionality is present (Yermish 2010).

Multipotentiality (Jacobsen 1999b; Daniels & Piechowski 2009; Webb et al. 2016; Heylighen, n.d.a; n.d.b): With their numerous interests and ability to do many things well, very high-IQ individuals crave stimulation and novelty and can get bored quickly (Lovecky 1986). This can make it difficult for them to choose a path, or stick to something and follow it through, which can be bewildering and frustrating for others (Nauta & Corten 2002).

Speed (Jacobsen 1999b; Streznewski 1999; Webb et al. 2016; Heylighen, n.d.a, n.d.b.): Thinking and speaking quickly, with rapid learning and mastery of new concepts, causes problems when others cannot keep up. Misunderstandings arise when, for example, others assume that such a person could not possibly, in the time available, have already thought through something properly or taken it seriously.

Charlton (2009) suggests that high IQ brings with it a tendency to over-use general intelligence, thereby overriding the instinctive and spontaneous forms of evolved behaviour which could be termed "common sense". What this means is that such "clever sillies" (Charlton 2009) rely on the use of abstract analysis even in situations such as social ones where this is not called for, resulting in socially inappropriate behaviour. As Kanazawa (2012) puts it, they rely on *thinking* in situations where they should be *feeling*.

Whilst these individual differences can cause confusion and difficulty with getting on smoothly or constructively with others, at worst they can engender actual hostility. Hostility from the high-IQ individual towards others can arise when others are experienced as frustrating and obstructive. Hostility towards high-IQ individuals can be a response to such individuals' own challenging behaviour (Falck 2013). Alternatively, hostility towards high-IQ individuals can derive from intolerance of exceptions (Webb et al. 2016) – others reacting negatively to difference – or from others feeling insecure and threatened (Falck 2013). In my research a main reason perceived by high-IQ individuals for others being hostile or obstructive was their envy of what was perceived as the high-IQ individual's advantage (Falck 2013). This – as explicated in the previous chapter – can lead to overt envious attacks or the more insidious *Schadenfreude*.

Nature of the difficulty: two main kinds

In the well-known originally Danish story *Keiserens nye Klaeder* (Andersen 1837), two tailors set out precisely to denigrate someone who could be envied for his position of advantage – an emperor who happens to have a weakness for fabulous clothes. They offer him what they promise will be the best garment ever, woven of unique thread that is invisible to anyone who is unfit for his position or stupid. When the emperor is undressed to fit the garment on, the tailors make a great show of adjusting it on him. To himself, however, he still looks naked. But he goes ahead with the public procession arranged to show off his new clothes. As neither he, nor anyone in the crowd of onlookers, wants to be judged stupid (demonstrating the importance within that society of intelligence), they all mimic each other in voicing their admiration of clothing that they cannot see. Amidst all of this a small child suddenly exclaims in amazement that the emperor is actually wearing nothing. The emperor hears this but ignores it and continues strutting along as though the nakedness that he fears might indeed be true has not been suggested.

One of my research interviewees brought up this story in the course of explaining what she saw as the root of the interpersonal difficulty she had suffered:

> It's like the emperor's child, the emperor's clothes, the child doesn't want to tell other people they are stupid, he just says the emperor is naked, and I think when you grow up as a gifted child and people not recognising that, which happened to me, maybe that's why I'm so aware of that, is they get irritated by that and they push it down, which happened to me …
>
> *(Ana)*

In contemplating this, I thought that it might well be that an extremely intelligent person can be like the small child in this story, as such a person has much more of a tendency to speak their mind, candidly saying the truth as they see it, and to act independently, not honouring group rules and sensibilities (Favier-Townsend 2014:62). This frequently triggers unfavourable reactions.

In my research interviews a great many more experiences of this kind were described. These involved the interviewee behaving spontaneously in an innocent, guileless way, and then being surprised to discover that others had taken offence. This demonstrated an essential naivety with regard to what others might expect, how they might be feeling, and how they might be predicted to experience and react to something. For example:

> I'd like to think that I'm generally a nice guy, but I can, involuntarily, hurt people by saying something or doing something or reacting in a certain way that is just not appropriate given their current state of mind. And that is something that happens to me time and time again.
>
> *(Hans)*

> I say stuff which makes people's hair go up on end …
>
> *(Jane)*

> … when it comes to politics, knowing what to say to whom and the implications of it, I was saying to a friend, I said, "I'm intelligent and therefore I feel I should be good at politics, but it's not an instinct". My friend, she said, "It's an instinct, politics, you don't necessarily have to be intelligent for it, you just know what to say, what not to say, when to

hold your tongue, when to speak, and there are people who are very good at making alliances and networking". I'm bad at it, I'm just bad ... I think I'm bad at it because – I can't put my finger on it ... I think I lack a certain understanding of what it is ...

(Jane)

As these experiences of behaving in a way that stumbles unawares into social transgression were similar to the child's behaviour in the above story, I categorised this prominent order of interpersonal difficulty as the "Naive Child" profile.

However, I then thought about how a high-IQ person can also behave like the emperor in the story. Extremely intelligent children will usually come to be aware of their intellectual advantage in relation to others (see Chapter 4), and – like the emperor – can accordingly become accustomed to and expectant of others' admiration. This can continue into adulthood, such as this experience interviewee Tracy described:

> I mean within two weeks of me starting my job ... it felt like ... I went home and I explained it like I was the messiah, like it was the second coming, because every meeting that I went into, they were just like, "Oh god we've been waiting for somebody like you [Tracy], we're so happy".

This is redolent of Tom Hayes's "God syndrome". Such treatment can create in such a person a confidence in their own abilities – even to the extent that they believe they are always right (as interviewee Wayne described in Chapter 3) – together with a frustration or impatience with what is experienced as others' slowness and/or incompetence. At worst, regularly experiencing such frustration can develop in the high-IQ person a derogatory attitude towards others, and this looks arrogant:

> ... people are idiots and they can't see what's in front of them. You have to spell it out for them.
>
> *(Harry)*

> Well, it's very difficult to respect authority if authority really clearly has no idea what it's doing. I have very low tolerance for ineptitude ... I've learnt to temper it in most situations, but I really do sometimes lose my rag completely when I see someone just blindly doing something because that's what they've been told to do, even if it makes no sense at all.
>
> *(Helene)*

> I know I'm a bit easy to draw judgement on people sometimes and that's a bias I have, so I think whenever I hear someone is talking about something that I would label as stupid things, then I just think oh god this

person must be, I don't know, someone I couldn't stand, and I think if they can enjoy this outside of work they just can't be clever enough to be able to do any positive contribution to whatever we do here.

(Max)

I initially tried to help her, but I became impatient and the feedback, my friend overheard the conversation, and said to me, "You know, what you do, you make people feel stupid." Yeah, and I think he was right. Yeah. I was impatient with her and I didn't help matters the way I approached it. I made her feel just bad.

(Hans)

[Speaking of her CEO] He is clearly someone who can't see what's going on … and maybe he just needs to be told, you know like, if he can't see what's going on. I mean, he's probably a bit, you know, stupid …

(Tess)

I categorised the above kinds of interpersonal attitudes and behaviour as the "Arrogant Emperor" profile. A person who becomes identified with that aspect of their experience can become reliant for their self-esteem on preserving a beguiling sense of having superior capability. This can lead to even self-protectively ignoring evidence to the contrary – like the emperor does in the story when he keeps marching ahead intent on preserving his preferred image of himself as someone who is impressive to others, regardless of what the reality is.

In my analysis of my own research and the literature, I found that these two main orders of interpersonal difficulty – Naive Child and Arrogant Emperor – proved effective at encapsulating most of the social predicaments evident in the data, as summarised below.

The "Naive Child" profile

This involves the very high-IQ person experiencing an incapability of reading social cues and politics correctly, blurting things out honestly without cognisance of the interpersonal nuances present, and not having awareness of others' psychological processes or being able to tune into these accurately. There is no hostility towards others, but they find themselves relationally "out of sync" with others, where things socially do not "click" or "flow" well. An example is a client of mine who said to me "I am the iceberg": he explained that when he arrives in a social situation, his presence seems to cause the conversation that was happily going along before his arrival to crash. Relevant examples from the literature on giftedness are as follows:

- Experiences of misunderstandings, confusions, friction, and unintended offences (Falck 2013).

- Receiving complaints of being too serious, sensitive, intense (Jacobsen 1999b; Daniels & Piechowski 2009; Webb et al. 2016).
- Having strong reactions even to things the other might not have seen as important or extreme (Grobman 2009; Falck 2013; Nauta & Ronner 2013; Fonseca 2016; Webb et al. 2016).
- Expecting others to keep up with their speed and efficiency and not understanding why they don't (Nauta & Corten 2002; Falck 2013; Webb et al. 2016).
- Not complying with social etiquette (Grobman 2006; Corten et al. 2006) because of not being aware of it. Not very diplomatic or tactful, not "saving another person's face" (Corten et al. 2006). Asks embarrassing questions (Heylighen, n.d.b).
- Strong content focus and can ignore social context (Corten et al. 2006). Task-oriented to the neglect of office politics, dress, and grooming (Webb et al. 2016).
- Being bad at socialising small talk (Corten et al. 2006; Falck 2013; Webb et al. 2016).

The "Arrogant Emperor" profile

Here the extremely intelligent person experiences feelings of impatience, frustration, and arrogance, sees others as slow or stupid, and accordingly exhibits challenging behaviour – including hostility – towards others. Being treated as the "oracle" (Erik) or "messiah" (Tracy) can contribute to this. An example is a client of mine who spoke of how, when he was performing on stage and had fans screaming their near-worship of him, he experienced feelings arising in him of despising their inane behaviour. It is also this profile that leads to the sorts of criminal daring described in Chapter 4. Relevant examples from the literature on giftedness are as follows:

- Showing boredom, frustration, impatience with others (Lovecky 1986; Jacobsen 1999b; Streznewski 1999; Falck 2013; Webb et al. 2016).
- Annoyance at others seeming slow and uncaring about quality (Jacobsen 1999b; Streznewski 1999; Falck 2013; Webb et al. 2016).
- Being critical of others (Grobman 2006; Falck 2013; Nauta & Ronner 2013). Intolerant of others' needs if they regard these as superficial (Lovecky 1986). Can use advanced vocabulary to "beat up" others with words (Webb et al. 2016:270).
- Challenging others (Falck 2013). Not listening to/accepting what others say (Nauta & Corten 2002). Being argumentative, questioning (Netz 2014; Webb et al. 2016).
- Obstinately wanting own way, insisting on being right and being in control (Falck 2013; Nauta & Ronner 2013; Webb et al. 2016). Being opinionated and stubborn rather than co-operative; reluctant to compromise (Heylighen, n.d.b).

- Not respecting authority/status: questioning of rules/authority, non-conforming (Falck 2013; Webb et al. 2016; Heylighen, n.d.b). What Lovecky (1986) calls "divergency".
- Being manipulative, exploiting own power (Maupin 2014; Webb et al. 2016).

Differences and connections between the two profiles

Table 5.1 directly compares and differentiates Naive Child versus Arrogant Emperor aspects of interpersonal relating.

One could ask whether there is any worthwhile rationale for creating designations like "Naive Child" and "Arrogant Emperor". The point is that they can usefully account for large categories of data, as shown above. They qualify for Charmaz's (2014:248) definition of what theoretical concepts are, in that they "subsume lesser categories with ease and by comparison hold more significance [and] account for more data". However, by using the Child and Emperor designations I open myself to the same problems that the entering of any "naming" territory encounters, such as the question of who fits which designation exactly, and what about cases where features of different designations seem to be

TABLE 5.1 Distinguishing Naive Child versus Arrogant Emperor characteristics of interpersonal relating

Naive Child	Arrogant Emperor
Naive, wondering, curious.	Arrogant, presumptuous, entitled.
Asking a lot of naive questions.	Making a lot of knowing criticisms.
Making factual "discovery-type" observations.	Making disparaging "already-informed" evaluations.
Not following established social rules because of not having awareness or understanding of what these are.	Not following established social rules because of deriding these and thinking you're above them.
Being immune to embarrassment/deference.	Being very sensitive to issues of ego/status.
A guileless blurting out driven by the inability to hold back the urgency of wanting to say something.	An impatient interrupting of others driven by viewing others' contributions as being less important than your own.
Being tactless out of innocence, not being able to perceive or predict how another will be affected.	Being tactless out of frustration/irritation/anger, not caring how another will be affected.
Attitude of having no personal expectations.	Attitude of expecting you are owed certain attentions and privileges.
Experiences – and stirs in others – bewildered awkwardness/discomfort.	Experiences – and stirs in others – defensive/attacking indignation.

simultaneously present? So it is important to emphasise that I am not using these concepts as rigid categorisations of people. Instead I am using them as metaphors that provide a shortcut way of grouping together, and referring to, clusters of specific related interpersonal attitudes, behaviours, and experiences. The same person could display elements of Child or elements of Emperor at different times. For example, interviewee Don described himself as being arrogant (Emperor), but he also described how others seemed to understand socialising in a way that he didn't (Child), and that he had had to set about trying to deliberately learn what to others appeared to come naturally.

In my research it appeared that in different individuals one or the other profile tended to be dominant – for example, interviewee Jane was predominantly Child, and interviewee Harry was predominantly Emperor. However, it could be that Harry's Emperor behaviour had been formed as a defence against the helplessness, confusion, and distress he felt as a Child: he had said that people thought of him as odd, and that he hated being set apart as different but couldn't help it, that the view others had of him was "He's an outsider, he's not like us …". Also, one could lead to another. For example, the genuinely innocent question of the Child could cause a bad reaction in another person who becomes obstructive or hostile and then the Child gets frustrated, angry, and treats the other person as though they're stupid, at which point the Child is behaving like an Emperor. The nature of these two profiles – and the similarities and differences between them – will be further elaborated in the next chapter.

Consequences of interpersonal difficulties

The discomfort and even hostility that interpersonal difficulty produces has varying degrees of impact on how extremely intelligent persons feel about themselves and others, and consequently upon the way they behave. Difficulties of this kind can lead to compounding intrapersonal and interpersonal repercussions in the following ways, which are ordered to show how such difficulties can sequentially lead a very high-IQ person to being in a situation that gets worse and worse:

a) *Feels different*, out of step with others, sense of alienation and aloneness (Streznewski 1999; Grobman 2009; Heylighen, n.d.b).
b) *Experiences awkward social interactions* through not communicating effectively with others (Corten et al. 2006; Fonseca 2016) and being misunderstood by others (Heylighen n.d.a; n.d.b).
c) *Difficulty fitting in* (Nauta & Ronner 2013; Fonseca 2016). Experiences of not feeling comfortable with others, and of being disliked and excluded, rejected (Lovecky 1986; Falck 2013).
d) *Regular conflicts with others* (Corten et al. 2006).
e) *Experiencing hostility from others*. Feeling disliked, even hated, and/or excluded. This includes unfriendly body language (e.g. "a cold stare"), negative reactions

(e.g. "get[s] my colleagues' backs up"), being "an object of ridicule", others being "closed off" to you, and having "made enemies" (Falck 2013).

f) *Being obstructed by others* – being prevented from utilising their abilities and making a contribution (Falck 2013), for example not being given job opportunities, visibility, or promotions.

g) *Being bullied* (Fonseca 2016). This can include mild experiences of teacher put-downs in class (Freeman 2010) and mocking parental comments like, "If you're so gifted why did you forget your lunch?" (Webb et al. 2016:269). More severe is being taunted with names used in a derogatory way such as "smart arse", "clever clogs", "know-it-all" (Falck 2013). And most extreme is actual violence, such as being beaten up.

h) *Feeling bad about self*. Experiencing things with others not going well, or being bullied, can lead to feeling there is something wrong with themselves, underrating themselves (Powell & Haden 1984; Heylighen, n.d.b), and developing low self-esteem (Webb et al. 2016).

i) *Withdrawing from others* because of the frustration of not having constructive communication with others (Corten et al. 2006). Withdrawal can also arise out of fear of failure, fear of others' envy, and feeling strange/different (Corten et al. 2006; Grobman 2006). Gifted individuals have been associated with being introverted (Lovecky 1986; Heylighen, n.d.b) and showing an avoidant attachment style (Falck 2013). In the workplace, those with an avoidant attachment style did less socialising than others, preferred being physically positioned at some social distance, and didn't seek social involvement (Falck 2013). In a study by Kaufmann (1992), 67% of gifted adults reported no participation in social activities outside work.

j) *Becomes isolated*, not belonging, feeling others are against them (Hollingworth 1942; Nauta & Ronner 2013), and staying away from others – what Persson (2009:5) calls "voluntary marginalisation".

The above consequences lead in compounding degrees to ostracism, which – as shown in Chapter 3 – is painful, and over time a lack of belonging is associated with many physical and psychological ill effects.

Impact on individuals' prospects of actualising their potential

The kinds of interpersonal difficulty detailed above can have a considerable impact on extremely intelligent individuals' prospects of actualising their potential. Towers maintains that those with IQ above 145 will often require special attention "if they are to make the most of their gifts" (1987:1). The following are further mentions of how relational issues interact with and affect the process and prospects of actualising high ability:

a) *Unable to find a channel for using abilities* (Streznewski 1999), as ways of utilising abilities always involve relating with others (Falck 2016).

b) *Restricts own learning* as a way of trying to resolve inner conflicts about their giftedness (Grobman 2009:112) – to be differentiated from a "true neurologically based learning disability".
c) *Limits performance* out of guilt at having higher ability than others (Grobman 2006).
d) *Gives up* on passion and ideals – "hides gifts" – so as to fit in, what Kerr & Cohn (cited in Webb et al. 2016:276) term "deviance fatigue".

From this it is apparent that in addition to extremely intelligent individuals perhaps encountering ways in which difficult social interactions limit their prospects of using their abilities, they may themselves seek to avoid difficult social interactions by restricting or giving up on their abilities. This was mentioned at the end of Chapter 4, as high-IQ individuals hiding themselves. Coleman (2012) found that the strategy most frequently employed by gifted youth for coping with social difficulty was that of "making themselves invisible".

Reasons for the stereotype

Based on all that has been presented above, it can be concluded that this extent of documented interpersonal difficulty is what has brought about the stereotype of social ineptness in relation to extreme intelligence. However, what purpose might such a stereotype serve?

Roland Persson's (2009) work on "the unwanted gifted and talented" considers the paradox of what is evidently both the desirability and undesirability of extreme intelligence. Whilst high potential and achievement can be pursued and admired, individuals who manifest high ability can also – as we have seen – often be subject to prejudice and bullying. Persson maintains that when gifted individuals create products or provide services (such as scientists, engineers, and industrial designers do) that are valued within their sociocultural context and thereby achieve the maintenance of existing social structures, or when they provide entertainment (such as sports figures, musicians, writers, and actors do), then such individuals are admired, supported, and encouraged. However, when a highly intelligent person is seen to be presenting a threat, which often means a threat in terms of bringing about change to familiar or preferred social structures and/or challenge to the currently held positions of dominance within that structure (threatening others' privilege, power, and influence), this threat is defended against by stigmatising the person who is posing the risk. Such threat can be experienced and reacted to with stigmatisation in contexts as varied as a junior school playground or a country's political regime. Stigmatisation means someone being devalued and overall dehumanised in the eyes of others, in a way that elicits emotional reactions such as pity, anger, anxiety, or disgust (Crocker & Quinee 2003). Persson sees stigmatisation as a way of trying to neutralise the impact that an extremely intelligent person can have. One of the examples he gives is of how Nelson Mandela was vilified within the country to whose existing social structure he was posing a threat (by those in power and their proponents), whereas outside of that country he was more uniformly hailed as an admirably gifted leader.

When presenting at the SENG (Supporting the Emotional Needs of the Gifted) conference in Denver, Colorado, I attended a session conducted by American psychotherapist Lisa Erickson who specialises in working with giftedness. She titled her session "Coming out Gifted as an Adult", and applied Steele's (1997) work on stereotype threat to "the phenomenon of adults minimizing, forgetting or denying [their] giftedness" (SENG 2015:20). The negative stereotypes about high-IQ individuals as being achievement-driven and socially inept will influence how such individuals feel about themselves, how they interact with others, and how they perform. I see this as producing a kind of "giftophobia", making high-IQ individuals prone to hiding themselves. As Tannenbaum (1983) asserted, some gifted individuals would rather underachieve and be popular than achieve high performance status and be socially ostracised. This has been confirmed in Cross et al.'s (1993) research on the social cognition of 1,460 gifted adolescents, which showed that such individuals wanted to have "normal" social interactions, that they believed they were treated differently when others were aware of their giftedness, and that they realised they could influence how others interacted with them by manipulating the information others have about them.

Although giftedness/high IQ is not listed as one of Moodley & Lubin's (2009) "big seven stigmatised identities", I would argue that it should be added, given how controversial an identification of or acknowledgment of high ability clearly is. Chaudoir & Fisher (2010) write about the complexity involved in making a decision about whether or not to reveal a concealable stigmatised identity. Their work certainly fits well with the documented ambivalence about recognising and accepting extreme intelligence and about "coming out gifted" (e.g. Lind 2000), although Chaudoir & Fisher (2010) do not mention giftedness as one of the identities to which their work could relate. They cite the motivations for disclosure of a concealable stigmatised identity as including a wish to alleviate inhibition and receive social support. The feared impact of disclosure includes the risk of becoming a target of prejudice with an outcome of social rejection and discrimination.

Summary

This chapter has further examined the social predicaments associated with extreme intelligence. It has been analysed how such difficulty arises, its nature, its consequences, and its impact on high-IQ individuals' prospects of actualising their potential. It has been shown how I have come to conceptualise the interpersonal difficulty as being of two main orders, which I have termed Naive Child and Arrogant Emperor. How these are distinguished from each other has been addressed, as well as their possible consequences such as stigmatisation, marginalisation, and stereotype threat.

I do not maintain that the kinds of interpersonal difficulties presented in this chapter are exclusive to very high-IQ individuals: these can arise amongst any human beings in different ways and to different degrees. However, with extremely intelligent individuals there is a predominance of certain kinds of experience because of their typical characteristics, and that has formed my focus. Neither do I maintain that all high-IQ people experience these problems. For those who do experience them, my interest is in how they arise and are perpetuated, and how they can be overcome. I am also interested in what makes the difference for high-IQ individuals who do not experience – or who have ceased to experience – such problems.

In the literature I have reviewed above, I noticed that interpersonal difficulty is almost entirely presented in a positivistic, stimulus-response, kind of way, portraying gifted individuals as having certain qualities and certain problems with others as a result. Such presentations are usually purely descriptive, such as "Gets impatient with others' slowness". What is missing is attention to how extremely intelligent individuals are involved in constructing their interpersonal relations such as through imposing their internal worlds on external situations. These processes occur more unconsciously but also influence the outcomes experienced. The Psychodynamic and Systemic bodies of knowledge provide a language for these more hidden, harder to articulate nuances of interpersonal experience – or unconscious processes – but these are virtually unrepresented in the literature on high IQ/giftedness. This will be elaborated on in Chapter 7.

References

Andersen, H. C. (1837). *Keiserens nye Klaeder*. [online] Translated from Danish by J. Hersholt. (n.d.). Available at: www.andersen.sdu.dk/vaerk/hersholt/TheEmperorsNewClothes_e.html. [Accessed 11 September 2016].

Charlton, B. G. (2009). Clever sillies: why high IQ people tend to be deficient in common sense. *Medical Hypotheses*, 73(6), pp. 867–870.

Charmaz, K. (2014). *Constructing Grounded Theory*. (2nd ed.). London: Sage.

Chaudoir, S. R. & Fisher, J. D. (2010). The disclosure processes model: understanding disclosure decision making and postdisclosure outcomes among people living with a concealable stigmatized identity. *Psychological Bulletin*, 136(2), pp. 236–256.

Coleman, L. J. (2012). Lived experience, mixed messages, and stigma. In: T. L. Cross & J. R. Cross (Eds.). *Handbook for Counselors Serving Students with Gifts and Talents: Development, Relationships, School Issues, and Counselling Needs/interventions*. Waco, TX: Prufrock Press. pp. 371–392.

Corten, F., Nauta, N. & Ronner, S. (2006). *Highly intelligent and gifted employees – Key to innovation?* (English translation). Academic paper delivered in Amsterdam,

11 October 2006 at International HRD-conference. [online] Available at: www.triplenine.org/articles/Nauta-200610.pdf. [Accessed 12 June 2012].

Crocker, J. & Quinee, D. M. (2003). Social stigma and the self: meanings, situations and self-esteem. In: F. H. Heatherton, R. E. Kleck, M. R. Hebl & J. G. Hull (Eds.). *The Social Psychology of Stigma*. New York: The Guildford Press. pp. 153–181.

Cross, T. L., Coleman, L. J. & Steward, R. A. (1993). The social cognition of gifted adolescents: An exploration of the stigma of giftedness paradigm. *Roeper Review*, 16(1), pp. 37–40.

Daniels, S. & Piechowski, M. M. (Eds.). (2009). *Living with Intensity*. Tucson, AZ: Great Potential Press.

Detterman, D. K. (2014). You should be teaching intelligence! *Intelligence*, 42, pp. 148–151.

De Vellis, R. F. (2012). *Scale Development – Theory and Applications*. (3rd ed.). London: Sage.

Dijkstra, P., Barelds, D. P. H., Ronner, S. & Nauta, A. P. (2012). Personality and well-being: do the intellectually gifted differ from the general population? *Advanced Development*, 13, pp. 103–118.

Falck, S. (2013). *Attachment Styles and Experience of Workplace Interpersonal Relating in Intellectually Gifted Adults*. Unpublished Practice Evaluation Project (PEP) submitted in partial fulfilment of the requirements for the Doctorate in Psychotherapy by Professional Studies at Metanoia Institute/Middlesex University.

Falck, S. (2016). *Make the Most of Your Mind*. [members' magazine] Wolverhampton: Mensa.

Favier-Townsend, A. (2014). *Perceived Causes and Long Term Effects of Delayed Academic Achievement in High IQ Adults*. Unpublished PhD thesis, University of Hertfordshire, UK.

Fonseca, C. (2016). *Emotional Intensity in Gifted Students – Helping Kids Cope with Explosive Feelings*. (2nd ed.). Waco, TX: Prufrock Press.

Freeman, J. (2010). *Gifted Lives: What Happens When Gifted Children Grow Up*. London: Routledge.

Freeman, J. (2013). The long-term effects of families and educational provision on gifted children. *Educational & Child Psychology*, 30(2), pp. 7–15.

Grobman, J. (2006). Underachievement in exceptionally gifted adolescents and young adults: a psychiatrist's view. *The Journal of Gifted Secondary Education*, 17, pp. 199–209.

Grobman, J. (2009). A psychodynamic psychotherapy approach to the emotional problems of exceptionally and profoundly gifted adolescents and adults: a psychiatrist's experience. *Journal for the Education of the Gifted*, 33(1), pp. 106–125.

Guenole, F., Speranza, M., Louis, J., Fourneret, P., Revol, O. & Baleyte, J.-M. (2015). Wechsler profiles in referred children with intellectual giftedness: association with trait-anxiety, emotional dysregulation, and heterogeneity of Piaget-like reasoning processes. *European Journal of Paediatric Neurology*, 19, pp. 402–410.

Heylighen, F. (n.d.a). *Gifted People and Their Problems*. [online] Available at: https://talentdevelop.com/articles/GPATP1.html. [Accessed 4 February 2017].

Heylighen, F. (n.d.b). *Characteristics and Problems of the Gifted: Neural Propagation Depth and Flow Motivation as a Model of Intelligence and Creativity*. [online] Available at: www.researchgate.net/profile/Francis_Heylighen/publication/228916918_Characteristics_and_Problems_of_the_Gifted_neural_propagation_depth_and_flow_motivation_as_a_model_of_intelligence_and_creativity/links/0046352960e925f295000000.pdf. [Accessed 4 February 2017].

Hollingworth, L. S. (1942). *Children above 180 IQ: Their Origin and Development*. New York: World Books.

Hollway, W. & Jefferson, T. (2013). *Doing Qualitative Research Differently – A Psychosocial Approach*. (2nd ed.). London: Sage.
Ibbotson, E. (2010). *The Ogre of Oglefort*. London: Macmillan Children's Books.
Irvine, L. (2012). Foreword to the first edition. In: S. Turing (Ed.). *Alan M. Turing – Centenary Edition*. Cambridge: Cambridge University Press, pp. xiv–xxiv.
Isaacson, W. (2011). *Steve Jobs: The Exclusive Biography*. New York: Simon & Schuster.
Jacobsen, M.-E. (1999b). *The Gifted Adult*. New York: Ballantine Books.
Jones, T. W. (2013). Equally cursed and blessed: do gifted and talented children experience poorer mental health and psychological well-being? *Educational & Child Psychology*, 30 (2), pp. 44–66.
Kanazawa, S. (2012). *The Intelligence Paradox*. Hoboken, NJ: John Wiley & Sons.
Kaufmann, F. A. (1992). What educators can learn from gifted adults. In: F. Monks & W. Peters (Eds.). *Talent for the Future*. Maastricht: Van Gorcum. pp. 38–46.
Kaufmann, F. A. & Matthews, D. J. (2012). On becoming themselves: the 1964–1968 presidential scholars 40 years later. *Roeper Review*, 34(2), pp. 83–93.
Lind, S. (2000). *Identity issues in intellectually/creatively gifted people: the coming out process: Identity development in gifted/gay students*. Paper presented at the Henry B. & Jocelyn Wallace National Research Symposium on Talent Development, Iowa City, IA.
Lopez, V. & Sotillo, M. (2009). Giftedness and social adjustment: evidence supporting the resilience approach in Spanish-speaking children and adolescents. *High Ability Studies*, 20(1), pp. 39–53.
Lovecky, D. V. (1986). Can you hear the flowers singing? Issues for gifted adults. *Journal of Counselling and Development*, 64, pp. 572–575.
Maupin, K. (2014). *Cheating, Dishonesty and Manipulation: Why Bright Kids Do It*. Tucson, AZ: Great Potential Press.
Moodley, R. & Lubin, D. B. (2009). Developing your career to working with multicultural and diversity clients. In: S. Palmer & R. Bor (Eds.). *The Practitioner's Handbook: A Guide for Counsellors, Psychotherapists and Counselling Psychologists*. London: Sage. pp. 156–157.
Nauta, N. & Corten, F. (2002). Gifted adults in work (English translation). *Tijdschrift voor Bedrijfs- en Verzekeringsgeneeeskunde (Journal for Occupational and Insurance Physicians)*, 10 (11), pp. 332–335. [online] Available at: www.sengifted.org/archives/articles/gifted-adults-in-work. [Accessed 12 June 2012].
Nauta, N. & Ronner, S. (2013). *Gifted Workers Hitting the Target*. Maastricht: Shaker Media.
Neihart, M. (1999). The impact of giftedness on psychological well-being: what does the empirical literature say? *Roeper Review*, 22(1), pp. 10–17.
Neihart, M., Reis, S. M., Robinson, N. M. & Moon, S. M. (Eds.). (2002). *The Social and Emotional Development of Gifted Children: What Do We Know?* Waco, TX: Prufrock Press.
Netz, H. (2014). Disagreement patterns in gifted classes. *Journal of Pragmatics*, 61, pp. 142–160.
Persson, R. S. (2009). The unwanted gifted and talented: a sociobiological perspective of the societal functions of giftedness. In: L. V. Shavinina (Ed.). *International Handbook on Giftedness*. Quebec: Springer. pp. 913–924.
Peyre, H., Ramus, F., Melchior, M., Forhan, A., Heude, B. & Gauvrit, N. (2016). Emotional, behavioural and social difficulties among high-IQ children during the preschool period: results of the EDEN mother-child cohort. *Personality and Individual Differences*, 94, pp. 366–371.

Powell, P. M. & Haden, T. (1984). The intellectual and psychosocial nature of extreme giftedness. *Roeper Review*, 6(3), pp. 131–133.

Rowling, J. K. (1997). *Harry Potter and the Philosopher's Stone*. London: Bloomsbury.

Ruf, D. L. (2009). *Five Levels of Gifted – School Issues and Educational Options*. Tucson, AZ: Great Potential Press.

SENG. (2015). *Soaring with SENG, Denver, Colorado*. [conference programme] Schenectady, NY: SENG.

Steele, C. M. (1997). A threat in the air: how stereotypes shape intellectual identity and performance. *American Psychologist*, 52(6), pp. 613–629.

Streznewski, M. K. (1999). *Gifted Grown Ups: The Mixed Blessings of Extraordinary Potential*. New York: John Wiley & Sons, Inc.

Tannenbaum, A. J. (1983). *Gifted Children*. New York: Macmillan.

Terman, L. M. (1925). *Genetic Studies of Genius, Vol.1: Mental and Physical Traits of a Thousand Gifted Children*. Stanford: Stanford University Press.

Towers, G. M. (1987a). The outsiders. *Gift of Fire*, 22. [online] Available at: www.cpsimoes.net/artigos/outsiders.html. [Accessed 5 February 2017].

Towers, G. M. (1987b). *IQ and the Problem of Social Adjustment*. [online] Available at: www.triplenine.org/Portals/0/Docs/download/IQ_and_the_Problem_of_Social_Adjustment.pdf. [Accessed 5 February 2017].

Vance, A. (2015). *Elon Musk*. London: Virgin Books.

Webb, J. T., Amend, E. R., Beljan, P., Webb, N. E., Kuzujanakis, M., Olenchak, F. R. & Goerss, J. (2016). *Misdiagnosis and Dual Diagnoses of Gifted Children and Adults*. (2nd ed.). Tucson, AZ: Great Potential Press.

Yermish, A. (2010). *Cheetahs on the Couch: Issues Affecting the Therapeutic Working Alliance with Clients Who are Cognitively Gifted*. Unpublished PhD thesis, Massachusetts School of Professional Psychology.

Zettergren, P. (2014). Adolescents with high IQ and their adjustment in adolescence and midlife. *Research in Human Development*, 11(3), pp. 186–203.

6

MADNESS, MISUNDERSTANDING, AND MISDIAGNOSIS

Is extreme intelligence a benefit or a liability?

> **Reflective Prompt 6:** If you were offered a completely safe procedure that would make you more intelligent than all other people, would you welcome such an outcome? In what ways do you imagine this could improve your life? Are there ways in which you believe it could make your life worse? How? If someone you loved was offered this procedure and you had to choose whether they would undergo it or not, what would your choice be? Why?

The concert is over. The hall is empty. But one member of the audience has stayed behind. Accomplished composer Hector Berlioz, who has just finished performing his *Symphonie fantastique*, notices this person. This is his description (Berlioz 1833):

> ... a man with long hair and piercing eyes and a strange, ravaged countenance, a creature haunted by genius, a Titan amongst giants ... the first sight of whom stirred me to the depths.

This person was Niccolò Paganini, another superlative musician – both composer and the most celebrated violin virtuoso of his time. Berlioz's words evoke the not uncommon image of exceptional talent causing torture, and his words also depict the strong reaction that can be felt when encountering a person of such talent. We looked in Chapter 4 at how people react when they recognise extreme intelligence, and in Chapter 5 at associated social troubles. Building now on what was covered in those chapters, the current chapter examines how the predicaments connected with a person standing out as being exceptional can escalate from eccentricity and interpersonal difficulty into madness and psychiatric diagnosis – or can be mistaken for the latter.

Is having the highest possible intelligence best?

There is a general tendency to consider higher intelligence as an absolute positive: the website of The International Society for Intelligence Research (ISIR) mentions that "the ultimate goal of all intelligence research is to understand how to increase intelligence". As seen in previous chapters, general intelligence – g – is the single measurable characteristic of individual difference that correlates with the greatest number of outcomes (Jensen 1998). For example, people with higher intelligence have better health and longevity even when socioeconomic variables are controlled for (Gottfredson & Deary 2004; Wraw et al. 2015), and higher self-control which is itself correlated with many positive outcomes (Meldrum et al. 2017). The traditional access routes into universities and high-paying occupations such as business and law rely on admission tests that advantage people with higher IQ (Sternberg 1995; Hunt 2011). For these reasons, intelligence remains a prized attribute. However, there is a point beyond which increased intelligence appears, paradoxically, to cease to lead straightforwardly to benefit: when entering the extreme intelligence range, things can start to look different. For example, recall the finding presented in Chapter 4 that criminality decreased with increasing measured intelligence but only until reaching the very highest level, where crime suddenly spiked (Schwartz et al. 2015; Oleson 2016). There is research showing that it is IQ near the top of the normal range that is most correlated with success in professional status and leadership. For example, a large-scale Swedish study showed that the average IQ score of CEOs was 115, which is one standard deviation above the norm (Adams et al. 2016). The cut-off point for this band of advantage is where the gifted range begins (i.e. at an IQ score of 130 and above). Managerial success has been shown to be lowest at the upper and lower IQ bounds (Ghiselli 1963a). Leaders are most successful when they have a higher IQ than their followers, but not too much higher: a 30 point difference causes the relationship either not to form, or to break up (Simonton 1984; 1985). Silverman (2013:86) writes about the "parallels at the extremes" of the Bell Curve: various problems such as social alienation and adjustment difficulties have been documented to affect individuals who fall within either extreme as compared with those within the mid-range majority. There are suggestions that the very fact of being extremely intelligent can impede a person's career progress (Lovecky 1986; Jacobsen 1999; Streznewski 1999; Corten et al. 2006; Persson 2009; Nauta & Ronner 2013). Very high IQ has also been documented as being a risk factor for mental disorder (MacCabe 2010; Weismann-Arcache & Tordjman 2012; Gale et al. 2013; Cross & Cross 2015; Karpinski et al. 2018). Rates of substance use increase in direct proportion to increase in intelligence (Kanazawa 2012). Why might this be?

We can approach answering this question by looking at a study that provides a notable exception to the above facts. The SMPY (Study of Mathematically Precocious Youth), introduced in Chapter 4, studied individuals with SAT-Math results that placed them within the top 0.5% of their age group (Hunt 2011). At 25-year follow-up the study participants had achieved way beyond the national average in successes such as high income and attaining doctorates, patents, and publications (Robertson et al. 2010). In addition, 2,385 of these study participants were divided into quartiles according to their results on that one SAT-Math test, and a striking finding was that on all professional success indices the graphs consistently show a steady increase in achievement going up through the 1st, 2nd, and 3rd quartiles, and then an even bigger surge in achievements in the 4th and highest quartile (Robertson et al. 2010). This showed that even within this group of exceptionally high test-scorers, those with higher scores consistently outperformed those with lower scores. However, something that significantly distinguishes this prospective longitudinal study is that its originator Professor Julian Stanley set out not only to select young individuals of extreme intelligence and then observe how they performed over time, but he also set out to enhance such performance: study participants were specifically nurtured intellectually so as to boost their chances of fulfilling their potential, so that they could "change the world" (Clynes 2016:153). One of the enrichment programmes providing such nurture was at the Johns Hopkins University's Centre for Talented Youth, and an example of a young adolescent who passed through this centre is founder of Facebook, Mark Zuckerberg (Clynes 2016), who, it can be argued, has indeed changed the world.

The achievements evidenced by the SMPY participants after receiving support to fulfil their potential, together with the data presented above on highest-IQ groups not necessarily faring very well, compellingly draw attention to the question of how characteristics associated with extreme intelligence are responded to and what impact this has on outcomes. For example, typical gifted/high-IQ traits include openness to experience and need for stimulation (Webb et al. 2016): it is easy to see that if these needs are not satisfied through worthwhile educational and occupational channels then the satisfying of them could be pursued through experimentation with drugs, making sense of the higher levels of drug use in this population. Enriched programmes for talented youth provide the participants not only with intellectual engagement but also with access to peers similar to themselves: when extremely intelligent individuals cannot find belonging with similar peers they have been documented to turn to using alcohol and other substances to dull their difficult feelings of being different, or to try to fit in more with dissimilar others (Webb et al. 2016). Once substance abuse becomes established the powerful physiological changes of addiction can set in and dictate the person's subsequent trajectory through life, which often spells the end of further prospects for actualising potential because the compulsions and associated lifestyle disruptions of addiction cycles are generally ruinous for the sustained focus, discipline, and perseverance required for reliable high achievement. It is clear that the heightened sensitivities of "hyper brain, hyper body" (Karpinski et al. 2018) can themselves become so difficult to live with if not appropriately supported that they might outweigh the kinds of advantages usually associated with higher intelligence.

Something that all the research is unequivocal about is that for very high IQ to lead to success, it is necessary for it to be paired with other supporting skills and traits. Professor Lewis Terman – who, starting in the 1920s, followed over 1,400 children of IQ 140 and higher (who came to be known as the Termites) for several decades in the first longitudinal study of its kind – also concluded that for the best outcomes, "exceptional ability required exceptional education" (Haier 2017:26). A study by Ghiselli (1963b) showed that people with higher intelligence get higher positions and more job success only when the higher intelligence is combined with supervisory ability, initiative, and self-assurance. This study was replicated 24 years later with the same results (Bowin & Attaran 1987). The importance of interpersonal competence and emotional intelligence – the ability to read and manage the emotions of self and others – for success and well-being at work for individuals, teams, and organisations has been well-established (Goleman 1998; Tan 2012). For example, Araoz (2007) researched which characteristics out of high IQ, relevant experience, and emotional intelligence, were most important for successful managers. He found that the highest rates of failure were in managers who were strong on the traditional combination of high IQ and relevant experience but had low emotional intelligence.

So, when people who have extreme intelligence do not succeed, is it only because of lack of adequate support to develop their potential and the necessary auxiliary skills, or could there be other factors at play?

Genius, madness, creativity

In *Touched with Fire* psychiatry professor Kay Redfield Jamison (1993) comprehensively studied the association since ancient times between distinguished creative accomplishment and problems with mental health. Something that is emphasised over and over again in the numerous sources she draws on, is that high intelligence, or "superior intellect" (William James, cited in Jamison 1993:54), is a necessary factor for such outstanding achievement. Jamison provides a detailed documentation of the remarkable frequency in highly creative individuals of mental health difficulties as evidenced by, for example, having been admitted to an asylum or psychiatric hospital and/or having attempted or completed suicide. She provides a list of names that is only a sample of such individuals but which itself fills three double-columned pages (1993:267). Examples she gives of famous poets, writers, composers, and artists so afflicted include, respectively, Sylvia Plath, Virginia Woolf, Robert Schumann, and Jackson Pollock. Simonton (2009) cites studies which show that relative to the general population, geniuses appear to exhibit a higher rate and intensity of psychopathology, and higher in proportion to the eminence of their work.

Overall, geniuses are about twice as likely to have lived through some mental or emotional difficulty, with depression being the most frequent, along with associated alcoholism and drug abuse (Simonton 2009). Jamison argues that the genesis of such problems can predominantly be attributed to manic-depressive illness, which I will here refer to by the name now used for this which is Bipolar Disorder. An updated suggestion that individuals with extremely high intelligence might be more prone to Bipolar Disorder is Gale et al.'s (2013) study of a very large sample of 1,049,607 Swedish men. Jamison (1993) documents that Bipolar Disorder has a strong genetic component (just like intelligence does) and that in fact both intelligence and Bipolar Disorder run in the same families. Simonton (2009) endorses this with several studies that suggest that psychopathology is more prevalent in families that produce geniuses. An example is that Charles Darwin and his cousin Frances Galton, both exceptional achievers, also both suffered a serious disorder at some point in their lives (Simonton 2009).

Simonton (2009) explains with his BVSR (Blind Variation Selective Retention) theory how, in order to create something new, thought processes are required that generate numerous ideational variations out of which – through a heuristic process of trial and error – the best ones eventually come to be selected and retained. The more ideational variations that can be generated, with speed and fluency, the more creative a person is. The variations generated can be blind (random, unknown, chaotic, unpredictable, serendipitous), or sighted (deliberate, rational, understood, controlled). This distinction can be exemplified in the very different processes of high mathematical ability that were dominant in G. H. Hardy – who for most of his distinguished mathematical career was a professor at Trinity College, Cambridge – in comparison with Srinivasa Ramanujan, who in 1914 travelled from his humble origins in India to become Hardy's protégé. Ramanujan produced such astounding, inexplicable and intuitive insight into mathematics (blind variation) that he was described as not just a genius but a "magician" (Kanigel 1991:281). Hardy, in contrast, applied careful systematic rigour (sighted variation) in creating step-by-step mathematical proofs that complied with the accepted academic protocols – techniques of which Ramanujan had no knowledge or experience. Simonton (2009) points out that different domains of accomplishment differ as to whether they rely predominantly on blind or sighted variation. Generally, artistic creativity is more blind (particularly that of expressionistic, avant-garde, or romantic artists) whereas scientific creativity is more sighted (particularly within the hard sciences like physics and chemistry) (Simonton 2009). Which of these kinds of creativity recognised geniuses have been mostly involved in is strongly correlated with his or her proneness to "madness", with the rate and intensity of psychopathology being higher in domains that are based on blind rather than sighted variation.

In order to generate blind variations, a person has to be in a state that facilitates random, chaotic ideas to emerge that he or she may not understand or feel in control of. Loosening the controls of conscious, rational thinking aids such a capacity. One state that promotes a loosening of conscious controls is falling asleep, and it is from dreams that some famed geniuses derived their creations. For example, Ramanujan had dreams in which he saw drops of blood that heralded the Hindu god Narasimha and following which "scrolls containing the most complicated mathematics used to unfold before his eyes" (Kanigel 1991:281). Such inspiration can also come in a waking dream or reverie, such as in the visions poet William Blake famously experienced, or the way Mozart would hear whole symphonies in his head and then write them down. A more contemporary example is that of Tony Cicoria (see Chapter 2) who, following being struck by lightning, would hear music that he wrote down in compositions (Sacks 2007).

The powerful force of that lightning strike clearly altered Cicoria's brain. Haier (2017) explains that the looseness of making mental associations that is the mark of creativity is promoted by disinhibition of neural processes. Such an effect can also be achieved by imbibing disinhibiting substances, a relatively mild one being alcohol, the use of which creative writers, for example, have a well-documented strong association with (Simonton 2009). Disinhibition that occurs through frontotemporal dementia (FTD) has also in rare cases been documented to release a dramatic new creative ability, often artistic (Haier 2017). Disease – as well as alcoholism, drug use, and mental illness – much more often leads to cognitive deterioration and overall degeneration rather than to genius creativity. And this highlights the dangers involved: the torture of the tormented genius, I think, refers precisely to the difficulty of walking the line between these two possible outcomes.

In Hans Eysenck's model of three personality patterns, "psychoticism" is the pattern that is correlated with creativity (cited in Simonton 2009). Psychoticism involves an increase in traits that sustain originality such as independence and the capacity for defocused attention (Simonton 2009), and divergent rather than convergent thinking (Jamison 1993). How this can edge towards the risk of madness – psychosis – is articulated by Koestler (1971:316–317) with a vivid analogy:

> ... the creative act always involves a regression to earlier, more primitive levels in the mental hierarchy, while other processes continue simultaneously on the rational surface – a condition that reminds one of a skin-diver with a breathing-tube. (Needless to say, the exercise has its dangers: skin-divers are prone to fall victims to the "rapture of the deep" and tear their breathing-tubes off ...) The capacity to regress, more or less at will, to the games of the underground, without losing contact with the surface, seems to be the essence of ... any form ... of creativity.

The most advanced, and in evolutionary terms most recently developed, apparatus in the mental hierarchy is the prefrontal cortex. This is associated with what is termed secondary process thinking, which is logical, rational, consciously controlled, and operates verbally – functionality that is sited in the left hemisphere of the brain. The more primitive or primary process thinking is illogical, irrational, unconscious, and arises in images and intuitions – "gut feelings". Such functionality is sited in the right hemisphere of the brain, and constitutes the earliest mode of thought present in very young children (Schore 2016). What is crucial for outstanding creative accomplishment is to be able to engage in primary process immersion but then move from it into some form of secondary process capture and record-making of the jewels of the deep. Mozart had to not only have the dream, but also had to be able to write it down in intelligible musical notation, which requires discipline and relevant education. Genius cannot flower without the creative – even hypomanic – bursts that are experienced being later subjected to discipline, rationality, and sustained effort (a point emphasised in Jamison's book also). It is the maintaining of balance between these processes, and the capacity to combine them, that is crucial. Einstein maintained that "combinatory play seems to be the essential feature in productive thought" (Hadamard, cited in Simonton 2009:71). The PFIT neurological model of intelligence (see Chapter 2) highlights the importance for intelligence of the integration of different brain areas. The failure of such integration is seen in savants who have marked ability in one region but deficits in others so that they typically have low IQ and cannot even care for themselves (Haier 2017).

What we have seen in this chapter so far draws attention to the importance of being able to accurately identify abilities and vulnerabilities so that a person might be able to be appropriately responded to and supported to achieve the best possible outcomes. But accurate identification is not easy.

Misdiagnosis

To be able to choose the most appropriate response to a person we first need to know what it is we are looking at. As a child Elon Musk "seemed to drift off into a trance" (Vance 2015:31) so often, totally ignoring others even if they yelled at him, that his parents and doctors worried he might be deaf. We can now understand that these dreamlike states were manifestations of the powerful creative processes that he was inwardly absorbed in, but his external behaviour was not understood or readily tolerated by those around him. Doctors, psychiatrists, psychologists, teachers, and psychotherapists are rarely taught much or even anything at all about giftedness or how features associated with extreme intelligence might easily be mistaken for signalling conditions that are diagnosed as pathological. For example, not sustaining attention during school classes is a diagnostic criterion for Attention-Deficit Hyperactivity Disorder (ADHD), but attention will also not be sustained by a perfectly healthy but extremely intelligent child who is utterly bored in such classes.

The research and debate that goes into the designating of diagnostic categories for human behaviour is extensive (e.g. see Paris & Phillips 2013), and it involves a lot of subjective decision-making about where to place boundaries that is not an exact science and changes over time and across countries and cultures.

Disagreement continues even amongst expert clinicians (Rhode & Klauber 2004; Webb et al. 2016) as to how to view or define different categories. Webb et al. (2016) deal in detail with how giftedness/high-IQ relates to a range of psychiatrically diagnosable disorders including ADHD, OCD (Obsessive Compulsive Disorder), and Bipolar Disorder, in each case naming similarities and incompatible or contradictory features. Here I will focus only on two such diagnoses – Autism Spectrum Disorder and Narcissistic Personality Disorder – on the basis of these being the ones that emerged during my research as being associated respectively with the two main orders of interpersonal difficulty that I identified in extremely intelligent adults and which I conceptualised as Naive Child and Arrogant Emperor.

Naive Child and autism

Naivety can derive from simply not having learned necessary information, such as a child who by his or her youthfulness has not yet been exposed to certain social situations and has not had the opportunity to learn about how these work and how they should best be navigated. Or naivety can derive from such learning not having taken place because of a cognitive incapability of registering, processing, retaining, and applying the necessary information that there has already been sufficient exposure to in relevant situations. Learning about and gaining interpersonal fluency usually accrue to a person in the ordinary course of development. However, several of my interviewees described that they felt this had not occurred for them in the way they noticed it seemed to have done for others.

> For my particular case it's quite strange. I see people developing social skills naturally. For me they never came naturally …
>
> (Don)

Mei: … it's always in my head that I'm very aware I'm not good with people and I'd rather not be in that position but I just have to be in that position so I need to learn how to deal with that.
SF: *But what makes you say you're not good with people?*
Mei: I don't know, because something inside me, people see me differently … I'm not a big social person and I don't know how to. I'm friendly with people, people like me as a friend, but I'm not as close as how I see others can be really friends. Girls' chats, I don't have that ability.

Deficits or persistent difficulties in social imagination, communication, interpretation, and interaction (The National Autistic Society, n.d.), or what Wing (1988) termed the "triad of impairments" in socialisation, communication, and imagination, are the key features of functioning that would qualify a person for a diagnosis of Autism Spectrum Disorder (ASD) (American Psychiatric

Association 2013; World Health Organization 2018). Autism is classed as a developmental disorder (World Health Organization 2018), suggesting that something that is expected to have taken place in the ordinary course of development has not taken place. For example, prior to the age of four (Doherty 2009) a child's cognitive development has not yet matured enough for them to have achieved Theory of Mind, which is the ability to perceive others' perspectives, intentions, and beliefs (Baron-Cohen et al. 1985). For an autistic person, this ability never develops naturally (Baron-Cohen 1995). And if a person has not "grown up" in this expected way, they might manifest behaviour and functioning that is associated with being more childlike, such as interpersonal naivety.

Several of my research interviewees, in the course of spontaneously pairing giftedness with interpersonal difficulty and mentioning high-IQ individuals they had encountered who they saw as being socially strange, then said that they thought such people might have Asperger's syndrome. For example:

> He's very bright but very odd, I'm sure he's on the Asperger's scale, like a lot of Mensa members are. I don't know if you've noticed that, but a lot of Mensa members are borderline autistic I think. I go away with them every year on a weekend in *[location]* and about 100 Mensa members go and there's always a good five to ten you can pick out that are odd, which is quite interesting.
>
> *(Tracy)*

The term "Asperger's syndrome" originates from a 1944 article by Austrian paediatrician Hans Asperger (cited in Rhode & Klauber 2004). It followed one year after the first delineation – by Leo Kanner (Rhode & Klauber 2004) – of autism as a syndrome. Asperger's work only gained prominence nearly 40 years later when Lorna Wing (Wing 1981) published a similar description for the English-speaking world, stimulating much research and debate on what constituted a diagnosis of Asperger's syndrome and how this was similar to or different from autism (Rhode & Klauber 2004). The first time that Asperger's Disorder was listed as a diagnostic entity was in the fourth edition of the *Diagnostic and Statistical Manual of Mental Disorders* or DSM (American Psychiatric Association 1994). Nineteen years later, in the fifth edition (American Psychiatric Association 2013) it was removed as a diagnostic entity distinct from ASD. Similarly, it no longer exists as a diagnostic category separate from ASD in the eleventh revision of the *International Statistical Classification of Diseases* or ICD (World Health Organization 2018). However, "Asperger's" is a term that remains in wide use.

In my research interviews, and also in audience comments when I presented my work to Mensa members at the Wellcome Collection, London, and at Trinity College, Cambridge, comparisons were made between extreme intelligence and Asperger's syndrome. Webb et al. (2016:134) caution against the way that the label of Asperger's has come to be liberally applied colloquially to "anyone who is socially awkward, has difficulties reading interpersonal cues, or simply seems aloof in social situations". They stress that autism is a significantly impairing condition, and that an ASD diagnosis is only appropriate when the associated features are severe and sustained (Webb et al. 2016:134). However, the very fact that what is being referred to here is a spectrum and can refer to a range from more subtly nuanced symptoms to severe ones, undermines any ideal of clear precision in diagnosis. Nevertheless, I will mention a few of the main differences pointed out by Webb et al. (2016) between giftedness and ASD – but remembering that it is also possible for high IQ and ASD to be co-present.

Individuals with ASD – unlike individuals purely with high IQ – find eye contact anxiety-provoking and their natural tendency is therefore to avoid eye contact. If empathy with others is in evidence this rules out a diagnosis of ASD. Whilst giftedness and ASD are both associated with focusing intensely on particular special interests, individuals with high IQ and not ASD seek to share their interests with others, can generalise facts from one situation to another, and can participate in turn-taking in conversation and stop talking about a pet interest when they pick up that their listener has lost interest. Furthermore, ASD involves physical clumsiness; marked literal-mindedness; and difficulty with abstract ideas, unstructured situations, and changes in routine. In a high-IQ person without ASD, social interaction is fluent, reciprocal, and unproblematic when with others who share their interests.

To try to gain more understanding about how extreme intelligence and autism relate to each other I tried to meet with Professor Simon Baron-Cohen, Director of the University of Cambridge's Autism Research Centre, but he emailed me to say that he was too busy to meet. I consulted with Caroline Hearst of Autism Matters, who provides UK-based CPD (Continuing Professional Development) trainings in autism. She asserted that autism has nothing to do with IQ, and that gifted individuals who manifest features similar to those of autistic individuals do so simply because they are also autistic (Hearst 2016). Dr Anna Remington of CRAE (the UCL Institute of Education's Centre for Research in Autism and Education) told me that the main difference between autism and giftedness is in the "spikes" of brain functioning involved. She explained that this can be observed in discrepancies between scores in verbal and non-verbal IQ: in autism there is a peak in non-verbal intelligence and a trough in verbal intelligence, whereas in giftedness there are peaks in both (Remington 2017). None of this helps to explain why there has developed a social stereotype that associates extremely intelligent people specifically – as opposed to any other defined minority group – with autism-like features of social ineptitude. The only study I have seen that starts to address precisely this is by Crespi (2016) who cites genetic findings that indicate that alleles for autism overlap broadly with alleles for high intelligence. Although autism in 44–52% of cases (The National Autistic Society, n.d.) involves a learning disability (low IQ), the paradox that it also appears to be associated with high IQ can be made sense of by the hypothesis that autism involves enhanced, but imbalanced, components of intelligence (Crespi 2016). Such a hypothesis is supported by evidence that autism and high IQ share convergent correlates such as large brain size, increased sensory and visual-spatial abilities, enhanced synaptic functions, increased attentional focus, occupational interests in engineering and physical sciences, and high levels of positive assortative mating (Crespi 2016). Karpinski et al. (2018) also confirmed a higher incidence of ASD in a sample of 3,715 individuals with IQ of 98th percentile or higher.

The UK National Autistic Society's position statement on the causes of autism is that these are still being investigated (National Autistic Society, n.d.). Grandin & Panek (2014) assert that this question is extremely complex, and that a genetic variation that is found in one autistic child will be absent in another. Psychoanalytic contributions to trying to understand autism have centred on early parent-child intersubjective experiences (Rhode & Klauber 2004), not (more recently) to say that the quality of these *causes* autism, but by way of charting how these are different when autism is involved. What is described is that the autistic person does not gain from these intersubjective experiences an internalised function that contains and regulates the high arousal that comes from external stimulation and internal affect, and the autistic person therefore tries to regulate this by withdrawing, or overdeveloping one area of functioning, or seeking security from predictable material objects rather than from unpredictable other people. All of this thinking describes the need to create a barrier of some form that protects against overwhelming experience: Bick (1968; 1986) termed this a "skin"; Tustin (1981; 1990) a "shell", or "autistic armour"; Bettelheim (1967) a "fortress". Meltzer et al. (1975) also described autistic children's need to protect themselves from a "bombardment of sensa". This accords with work on the perceptual sensitivity and intensity in autism, such as the "Intense World" theory of autism (Markram & Markram 2010). It also accords with the convergent correlates of high IQ and increased sensory sensitivity found in Crespi's (2016) study mentioned above, and Karpinski et al.'s (2018) "hyper brain/hyper body" findings. Similarities are obvious here with the work on perceptual sensitivity and intensity in giftedness, such as Dabrowski's (1964) supersensitivities/overexcitabilities.

Hearst (2016) said that the intervention she knows of with autistic children that seems to be most effective, is that of the therapist participating in matching what the autistic child is doing: if the child is spinning or flapping, the therapist does the same. She says this calms the child, and then they can start to relate. Essentially this is an intervention that involves mirroring (see Chapter 3) and resonates with the work on how early intersubjective attunement (see Schore 2016) helps to regulate the child's emotions and build a sense of security. Hearst (2016) spoke of how autistic people have trouble self-regulating. This could arise because the required intersubjective experiences have not been available (which was the assumption of Leo Kanner whose 1943 work described autistic children's mothers as overly intellectual and cold emotionally, which led to the term "refrigerator mother" – cited in Rhode & Klauber 2004), or it could arise because the available intersubjective provision has been unable to be made use of in the usual way. Research using EEG and neuroimaging (cited in Mollon 2001:200) has found that "the mother's right brain regulates the infant's states of affective arousal through the medium of the infant's right brain". If the brain of an infant, or indeed mother, is "wired differently", might this process not be able to unfold in the usual way, leaving the emotional-intelligence-type functions that are associated with the right hemisphere of the brain underdeveloped? Kanner's observations of autistic children's mothers as overly intellectual could simply have been observations of the much more recently evidenced correlation between high intelligence and ASD reported above (with the old trap of correlation being mistaken for causation).

Steve Silberman's book *Neurotribes* (2015) highlights neurodiversity: he asks whether autism is a devastating developmental condition, a lifelong disability, or a naturally occurring form of cognitive difference akin to certain forms of genius. It is interesting that he, too, brings in the association with high IQ. People who comprise the ordinarily functioning non-autistic majority – and non-extremely-high-IQ majority – are termed "neurotypicals" or NTs. This brings up the question of how certain presentations of individual difference become classified as a disorder. Giftedness is not classified as a disorder. Would the implications of extreme intelligence as an individual difference that presents, for example, special educational needs, only become of mainstream concern if it were so classified? Homosexuality is an individual difference that was classified as a disorder in the DSM until it was removed in 1973. Hearst (2016) wants to see autism similarly removed from the DSM.

In my view the main point of this is: what is to be done about it? I believe ways of trying to delineate and understand these sorts of individual differences should primarily be in the service of informing choices that have to be made about how to optimally respond when aspects of experience and behaviour cause difficulty and distress because they are not ordinarily understood or catered for within the general day-to-day social systems in which they manifest. Webb et al. (2016) assert that what is required for autism is social skills training and what is required for giftedness is educational opportunities. If, however, a person is affected by both autism and high intelligence, he or she might need both interventions, and the social skills training would have to be particularly differentiated for high-IQ participants. For example, one of the people behind the UK-based website "The Hidden Aspie" (www.thehiddenaspie.com) approached me seeking training for high-IQ autistic adults who struggle with social interaction but who are too high-functioning for the social skills training resources that the UK's National Autistic Society provide such as their *Social Eyes* interactive programme supported by training manual and DVDs. A study has shown that high-IQ autistic people can learn to mask and adapt their social difficulties but it comes at a price of anxiety (Livingston et al. 2018).

Hearst (2016) does not want diagnosis for autistic individuals, just identification. She says the best "treatment" is for autistic people to meet others like themselves who they can talk with and relate to about their experiences and with whom they can feel that they have similarity. This links back with Chapter 3's theme of needing to belong. It also recalls the concepts introduced in Chapter 4 of homophily and twinship transference.

Arrogant Emperor and narcissism

In the course of my research I also encountered the label of "narcissism" being used in relation to my topic. For example, where I was doing my doctorate it was accepted that it could be difficult to recruit even single-digit numbers of research participants. When I presented that my first research call had received a few hundred offers of participation, the presiding member of the teaching staff immediately declared that these individuals were "flocking in their droves" to participate in my research so as "to have narcissistic gratification of their high IQ being recognised". This interpretation shocked me, as it demonstrated the marked compassion barrier mentioned in Chapter 4: in any other population group in psychotherapy research a high number of individuals volunteering to participate would be seen as evidence that the issue being researched (such as, say, gender dysphoria, or racial discrimination) is of salience to affected individuals. Having recognition of any minority experience is usually portrayed as being of value for affected individuals. However, where extreme intelligence is concerned the search for recognition and understanding was construed as a pursuit of "narcissistic gratification".

As with the colloquial use of the label of Asperger's, labelling someone as narcissistic is often freely done, in the latter case to describe behaviour that appears self-centred or arrogant. Such behaviour accords with my Arrogant Emperor profile. However, as with ASD, a diagnosis of Narcissistic Personality Disorder (NPD) is only appropriate when the associated features are severe and persisting. I will again mention a few of the main differences that Webb et al. (2016) point out between giftedness and narcissism – remembering again that it is also possible for giftedness and NPD to be co-present.

Individuals with NPD – unlike individuals purely with high IQ – have grandiose fantasies about, and seek, success only because of wanting admiration and prestige, not for the value or personal meaning of the activity involved. If actual exceptional competence and achievement are in evidence this rules out a diagnosis of NPD. Whilst in both giftedness and NPD haughtiness can be displayed, individuals with high IQ only – unlike those who have NPD – behave this way when faced with others' incompetence but can be humble when with intellectual equals (or superiors). NPD, as opposed to high-IQ alone, involves exploitativeness of others, a lack of empathy, and rage when gratification is not forthcoming. In a high-IQ person without NPD, an appearance of self-confidence is based on genuine strong self-esteem and belief in their own ability.

In NPD an appearance of self-confidence is an attempt to conceal a very fragile self-esteem and an underlying sense of deficiency.

Arrogance, like naivety, can also derive from not having learned necessary prosocial information. Freud (1914:90) maintained that we all begin life in a state of "primary narcissism" where our existence is centred on gaining satisfaction of our own needs and we are not aware of others' needs and do not make a contribution towards reciprocating to them the care they give us and the sacrifices they make for us. But we are meant to outgrow this selfish phase. If, however, a child is always treated as special and admired and indulged, they can fail to outgrow this self-centredness because they are continually being treated as royalty. They therefore continue as "His Majesty the Baby" (Freud 1914:91). Behaving in this Emperor-like way in contexts outside of the immediate family, at an age when others will expect such behaviour to have long ceased, will be sure to provoke interpersonal difficulty.

Horton (2011) presents empirical evidence for the Psychodynamic and Social Learning Theory explanations of how psychiatrically diagnosable narcissism develops. The Psychodynamic explanations are threefold. The first maintains that early care-giving that is excessively neglectful or traumatic can cause the child to retreat into a protective self-focus (Kernberg 1975, cited in Horton 2011): it is as though the child resorts to gazing at himself in an actual mirror in the absence of experiencing an effective relational mirror. The second Psychodynamic explanation is that early care-giving that is excessively pampering and overindulgent does not frustrate the child's primitive grandiosity and leaves the child carrying that unrealistic view of herself into adulthood (Kohut 1977, cited in Horton 2011). The third explanation is that narcissism is created by parents who strategically exploit the child to fulfil their own ambitions (Rothstein 1979, cited in Horton 2011). The Social Learning Theory perspective holds that children who are adored, indulged, and given few limitations and boundaries are taught that they are superior and entitled, and that others are inferior, weak, and easily manipulated (Millon 1981, cited in Horton 2011).

From these descriptions it is easy to see how the characteristics of extremely intelligent children can make them susceptible to any of these developmental trajectories. Parents who cannot relate to and engage with their child's intensities can leave the child feeling neglected, and parents who try to suppress the child's precocity – particularly if violently – cause trauma. Webb et al. (2016) write about how parents might stand back in awe of their gifted child rather than providing the guidance and boundaries needed, and might use giftedness to justify the excusing of bad behaviour. It is not uncommon for the toxic behaviour of adults also to be tolerated because of their talents being valued, even though toxic behaviour – particularly in leadership positions – has been evidenced to ultimately harm organisations (Kusy & Holloway 2009).

When a child manifests impressive abilities that attract attention and admiration it might be hard for proud parents not to be tempted to appropriate this to boost their own ambitions and self-esteem (encapsulated in the "Tiger

Mother" and "stage parent" stereotypes). This can also result in favouritism being shown towards a gifted child (Webb et al. 2016). A child who is admired for her abilities, which feel ordinary to her, can disrespect those who treat her as though she is exceptional, and may not be able to resist the temptation to use her abilities to manipulate others (see Maupin 2014). Miller's (1997) *The Drama of the Gifted Child* deals with what she calls the "vicious circle of contempt". A child who experiences others as slow and less capable than himself, could naturally come to view them as inferior, unless he can have his own experience understood and be helped to understand, respect, and appreciate diversity. High-IQ individuals who repeatedly get the message that they are seen as brilliant can develop expectations about what they should be entitled to, for example in terms of occupation or remuneration, and they can become correspondingly dissatisfied if things are not working out for them in that way. A person who behaves like this can appear narcissistic, but this needs to be differentiated from an actual diagnosis of NPD.

The DSM-5 recognises that "many highly successful individuals display personality traits that might be considered narcissistic", and that NPD is only diagnosable when these traits are "inflexible, maladaptive, and persisting, and cause significant functional impairment or subjective distress" (cited in Webb et al. 2016:114). Webb et al. (2016:113) describe a "healthy narcissism", and Grobman (2009) a "healthy grandiosity", where self-belief and self-absorption to a high degree – and even a willingness to disregard others when intensely focused on their own goals – are necessary for achieving the application and dedication needed to carry out demanding large-scale innovative projects and shift boundaries in disciplines. Superior confidence is necessary in surgeons and allied professionals for them to be able to bear the great responsibility of their jobs and exert tasks that involve exceptional skill and consequence for human life, but such confidence can be misconstrued as arrogance (Webb et al. 2016).

Aetiological similarities

Whilst Table 5.1 (in Chapter 5) specifies differences between the Naive Child and Arrogant Emperor profiles, there are some similarities in how they come about. Both profiles involve features that a child is expected to outgrow. Developing Theory of Mind (which fails to happen in autism), and relinquishing self-centredness (which fails to happen in narcissism), are prosocial developments that aid co-operation, community, and collaboration. Both the Naive Child and the Arrogant Emperor involve a difficulty in finding a comfortable place in relation to others, with effective intercommunication, and it is a difficulty that seems to be based in a deficit in empathy or what Fonagy et al. (2004) have defined as "mentalisation" – what is commonly described colloquially as "putting oneself in another's shoes". A failing in this could arise out of not (or perhaps not yet) having the capacity to do so, like a child who developmentally has not yet acquired Theory of Mind. Or it could arise from not being willing to and therefore refusing to put yourself in another's shoes because you are resolutely focused only on your own experience and wishes – such as the Emperor-like disdain of Marie Antoinette's famous "Let them eat cake". This deficit can also arise quite straightforwardly out of never having been alerted to the fact that putting yourself in another's shoes is something you could be doing that would be helpful to do. This could pertain to the Child or the Emperor, through a simple lack of information or psychoeducation. It could also apply to anyone at any point in time where they happen not to be being thoughtful or considerate, perhaps because of being in a state of high arousal themselves (such as being in a state of anger or distress) that makes them "selfish". Goleman (1998) terms this being "amygdala-highjacked" because it involves being unable to use the prefrontal cortex to regulate the visceral fight-flight response and be able to think, reason, and imaginatively enter into what another's experience might be like. An important point, however, in how this pertains to extreme intelligence, is that it is more difficult to put oneself in another's shoes the more that the other is different from oneself. And when an extremely intelligent person is in an environment in which he or she is for the majority of the time not being understood and satisfyingly connected with by others, such a person can be in a constant state of some degree of anger or distress and can be constantly trying to get his or her own needs met, and can therefore be particularly unavailable to empathising or mentalising with others. Research has shown that in gifted students, all dimensions of social skills correlate positively with empathy (Ishak et al. 2014).

Figure 6.1 represents how the best interpersonal relating is facilitated by a minimum of both naivety (Child) and arrogance (Emperor). It indicates that there is a range in acuteness of these ways of being, from the occasional manifestation to the more entrenched and through to clinically diagnosable proportions. The x axis represents a continuum of naivety from low to high, and the y axis represents a continuum of arrogance from low to high. With increasing naivety and/or arrogance in a person's interpersonal interactions, the shading increasingly darkens to represent the increasing difficulty of interpersonal relating. This diagram also represents the fact that high levels of interpersonal naivety can look like symptoms of autism, and high levels of arrogance can look like symptoms of narcissism, requiring alertness to the possibility of misdiagnosis. Of course, as described above, autism or narcissism can also be co-present with extreme intelligence. This diagram is for conceptual purposes only and in no way suggests that extreme intelligence *leads to* autism or narcissism.

It is a person who demonstrates the sort of social awkwardness of my Naive Child designation who has typically been called a "nerd" or a "geek", which are terms that several of my interviewees made reference to. The Oxford English Dictionary (Soanes et al. 2006) definitions of these and other similar words are as follows:

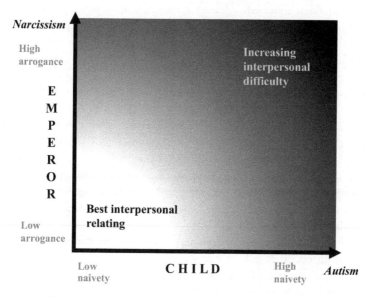

FIGURE 6.1 Child and Emperor: naivety and arrogance in interpersonal relating

Nerd: a foolish or contemptible person who lacks social skills or is boringly studious; a single-minded expert in a particular technical field.
Geek: an unfashionable or socially inept person; engage in or discuss computer-related tasks obsessively or with great attention to technical detail.
Dork: a contemptible, socially inept person.
Dweeb: a boring, studious, or socially inept person.

What these definitions have in common is that a person being studious and having technical expertise is linked with being boring as well as lacking in social skill, and is – and this is the most concerning part – *contemptible*. Why would such a person attract contempt? The example of usage that the Oxford English Dictionary gives for the word "contempt" is this: "This action displays an arrogant contempt for the wishes of the majority." This evokes my Arrogant Emperor designation. It appears that the sheer fact of being different, not the same as the majority, can be viewed as an act of arrogance or contempt for others and for how they feel or what they want, as though being different is received as an insult, and this in turn elicits contempt for such a person. Similarly, the word "prodigy" comes from the Latin *prodigium*, which means "a monster that violates the natural order" (Williams 2017). Recall Chapter 4's discussion of gifted individuals being "out of order" or "out of line". At bottom this returns to Chapter 3's theme of belonging within a group, and apprehending which individuals are adversaries or allies: those who share recognisable characteristics and behaviours – the similarities of homophily – are more easily recognised as allies; those who deviate are more readily perceived as adversaries. And groups exert strong controls to keep their members cohering: the word "contempt" is also what is used to denote lack of compliance with a nation's rules of law in the serious legal offence of contempt of court.

This brings us back to what I mentioned in Chapter 1 regarding the "hubris followed by nemesis" caution that is ubiquitous in myth and literature: do not defy the gods – "the gods" also being a society's authority figures, such as judges in courts of law and diagnosing psychiatrists. One can see why systems such as the DSM can be criticised as constituting a tool of social control: the diagnostic label of Pathological Demand Avoidance relates to a person not wanting to do what others want him or her to do; a diagnosis of Oppositional Defiant Disorder is again about opposing rather than complying with others; narcissism relates to having inflated belief in individual power; autism involves thinking differently from others. However, some form of social control is also required for achieving communal living. None of these diagnosable behaviours aid a social group in its task of maintaining its cohesiveness, which it does by augmenting its safe boundaries and seeking from its members obedience, co-operation, and adherence to – rather than challenges or threats to – the collective status quo. That is why groups engage in processes such as stigmatisation. It is the same conundrum that parents are facing when they resort to trying to subjugate their strong-willed gifted child. From this it becomes apparent how tendencies that have been identified as predominating in – and even being necessary to – genius, such as autonomy and non-conformity, are generally unsupported by the social systems around us and in ordinary daily life can be treated as problematic and even diagnosed as pathological.

Benefit, liability, and relational influences

We have been considering whether extreme intelligence is a benefit or a liability. But how we even define benefit or liability depends on what our underlying values are – for example, to create highly distinguished work, with the costs that exacts, or to lead a balanced life. However, it does appear that some element of liability is inherent within marked ability, given the genetic correlation evidenced between genius and psychopathology, but also, significantly, given the way that negative social reactions can cause distress. A gifted person's need to sequester themselves from company to preserve their independence of mind (Persson 2009) can make them susceptible to isolation. Neglect of their special educational needs or their dual or multiple exceptionality, and misunderstanding and misdiagnosis of their behaviour, plus the lack of acceptance and even strong resistance their originality might meet with, can take its toll on mental health. We all dread rejection. In addition, other prejudices can have a strong impact: for example, it is not Alan Turing's genius that tormented him but the way he was persecuted for his homosexuality.

Interpersonal relationships are key in affecting outcomes. Every young child has a core biopsychosocial drive to secure and deepen their attachment bond with a primary caregiver (see Chapter 3): when this drive is harnessed by an ambitious parent the child's wish to please the parent can become a cornerstone in their later achievement. There are many famous cases of this: Mozart had such a relationship with his intensely dedicated father. More modern examples in music include outstanding pop stars Michael Jackson and Britney Spears who each had a relentlessly pressurising parent. Examples in sport include champion golfer Tiger Woods and tennis champion Andre Agassi who were both initially coached by immensely zealous fathers (the "Tiger Mother" syndrome again). All of these relationships yielded benefit in stellar achievements, as well as liability in considerable intrapersonal and interpersonal disturbance.

Other parents can be instrumental in curbing their child's single-minded focus on a particular interest out of a belief that this is unhealthily unbalanced behaviour. It is true that obsessive dedication to work can entail sacrifice of the comforts and satisfactions of sustainable close relationships. For example, Ramanujan's commitment to pursue his intellectual development brought on years of separation from his young wife and close community, who, together with his pained mother, were left to celebrate at great distance, in India, the mark of his success in publications that he laboured on oceans away in Cambridge, England. He did of course have the *in situ* support of his mentor Hardy, and no genius succeeds in complete isolation without having at least collaborators or patrons. Often exceptional achievers have someone even closer – sometimes a spouse – who enables their work by providing extensive support in handling domestic, administrative, and publicity matters. Just two examples of such formative devotion include prize-winning poet Edna St Vincent Millay's husband Eugen Jan Boissevain and celebrated composer Edward Elgar's wife Caroline Alice Elgar.

Possibly even more important than providing these practical supports, is the emotional and psychological stability and security that an enduring attachment relationship can bring. Often the centrality is underestimated of relational processes in providing the motivation and regulation in a person's functioning. Intense love affairs have fuelled great works of art – one example being the great productivity Picasso was inspired to by, in particular, his mistress and muse Marie-Thérèse Walter (although he also created a trail of relational devastation). Long-term close relationships provide a secure base from which a person can engage in exploration of the world around them as well as exploration of their own intellect and creative powers. The primary caregiver – usually the mother – helps regulate an infant's states of distress when hungry, tired, overstimulated, or otherwise dysregulated, by offering not only material necessities but also soothing words and touch and a comfortingly familiar scent and presence. These early experiences of co-regulation come to be internalised and build the capacity for self-regulation. Co-regulation later continues in intimate personal relationships and is also provided in therapeutic relationships. Schore (2016) sees all mental health disorders as disorders of affect regulation. It has been well-evidenced that young children feel free and confident to engage in exploration in direct proportion to the safety and reliability of their secure base (e.g. see Cassidy & Shaver 2008). Even in adulthood the importance of a relational secure base cannot be underestimated: one striking example of the shock of its loss is how the brilliantly innovative and award-winning fashion designer Lee Alexander McQueen, CBE, at the age of 40 and at the peak of his extraordinarily creative career committed suicide on the night before his much beloved mother's funeral.

Summary

I can sum up the essence of this chapter with words adapted from *Star Trek: The Next Generation*: extremely intelligent persons will never come up against a greater adversary than their own potential. (This sage warning is spoken – in series 3, episode 1 – by eminent scientist Dr Paul Stubbs to the talented 17-year-old acting ensign Wesley Crusher who has caused serious risk to the whole starship by an accident with an experiment he was conducting.) In this chapter the risks associated with extreme intelligence have been considered, looking at paradoxical research on high IQ/giftedness being correlated with the highest of human achievement as well as with higher rates of career difficulty, mental illness, and substance use. Research on the higher incidence of autism in extremely high-IQ individuals has been considered. The neuropsychology of creativity has been discussed, explaining how the capacity for genius (an aspect of this being termed "psychoticism") can edge towards madness (psychosis). Misdiagnosis of giftedness has also been discussed, with a focus on the ways in which the Naive Child profile relates to autism and the Arrogant Emperor profile to narcissism. It has been explained how social systems' tendencies to pathologise and suppress non-compliance do not support the healthy development of genius with its essence of nonconformity. And it has been shown that although genius is empirically linked with madness, achieving genius is impossible without discipline, rationality, and sustained attention and effort. Robust self-regulation, with its roots in infant-caregiver co-regulation, and ongoing support in adult co-regulating relationships, helps contain the danger so as to facilitate distinguished accomplishment and avert self-destruction. The point has been made of the importance attachment relationships have in providing drive and succour for superlative achievement or becoming a catalyst in disturbance and despair. Famous cases of this have been given in music, sport, mathematics, poetry, art, and fashion. The lasting effects of early relational experiences will be explored in the next chapter.

References

Adams, R. B., Keloharju, M. & Knupfer, S. (2016). *Are CEOs Born Leaders? Lessons from Traits of a Million Individuals*. [online] Available at: https://papers.ssrn.com/sol3/papers.cfm?abstract_id=2436765##. [Accessed 26 March 17].

American Psychiatric Association. (1994). *Diagnostic and Statistical Manual of Mental Disorders: DSM-IV*. (4th ed.). Washington, DC: American Psychiatric Publishing.
American Psychiatric Association. (2013). *Diagnostic and Statistical Manual of Mental Disorders: DSM-5*. (5th ed.). Washington, DC: American Psychiatric Publishing.
Araoz, C. F. (2007). *Great People Decisions*. Hoboken, NJ: John Wiley & Sons.
Baron-Cohen, S. (1995). *Mindblindness: An Essay on Autism and Theory of Mind*. London: The MIT Press.
Baron-Cohen, S., Leslie, A. & Frith, U. (1985). Does the autistic child have a "theory of mind"? *Cognition*, 21, pp. 37–46.
Berlioz, H. (1833). *The Memoirs of Berlioz*. Translated from the French by David Cairns (1970). St Albans: Panther.
Bettelheim, B. (1967). *The Empty Fortress*. New York: Free Press.
Bick, E. (1968). The experience of the skin in early object-relations. *International Journal of Psycho-Analysis*, 49, pp. 484–486.
Bick, E. (1986). Further considerations on the function of the skin in early object relations. *British Journal of Psychotherapy*, 2, pp. 292–299.
Bowin, R. B. & Attaran, M. (1987). The Ghiselli study of abilities and traits of more and less successful middle managers: a replication. *Psychological Reports*, 60(3c), pp. 1275–1277.
Cassidy, J. & Shaver, P. R. (Eds.). (2008). *Handbook of Attachment: Theory, Research, and Clinical Applications*. (2nd ed.). New York: The Guilford Press.
Clynes, T. (2016). How to raise a genius. *Nature*, 537, pp. 152–155.
Corten, F., Nauta, N. & Ronner, S. (2006). *Highly intelligent and gifted employees – key to innovation?* (English translation). Academic paper delivered in Amsterdam, 11 October 2006 at International HRD-conference. [online] Available at: www.triplenine.org/articles/Nauta-200610.pdf. [Accessed 12 June 2012].
Crespi, B. J. (2016). Autism as a disorder of high intelligence. *Frontiers in Neuroscience*, 10. Published online: doi: 10.3389/fnins.2016.00300.
Cross, J. R. & Cross, T. L. (2015). Clinical and mental health issues in counseling the gifted individual. *Journal of Counseling & Development*, 93(2), pp. 163–172.
Dabrowski, K. (1964). *Positive Disintegration*. London: Little, Brown.
Doherty, M. (2009). *Theory of Mind: How Children Understand Others' Thoughts and Feelings*. New York: Psychology Press.
Fonagy, P., Gergely, G., Jurist, E. L. & Target, M. (2004). *Affect Regulation, Mentalization, and the Development of the Self*. London: Karnac.
Freud, S. (1914). On narcissism: an introduction. In: J. Strachey (Ed.). *The Standard Edition of the Complete Psychological Works of Sigmund Freud Volume XIV*. Reprint 2001. London: Vintage. pp. 67–102.
Gale, C. R., Batty, G. D., McIntosh, A. M., Porteous, D. J., Deary, I. J. & Rasmussen, F. (2013). Is bipolar disorder more common in highly intelligent people? A cohort study of a million men. *Molecular Psychiatry*, 18(2), pp. 190–194.
Ghiselli, E. E. (1963a). Intelligence and managerial success. *Psychological Reports*, 12(3), p. 898.
Ghiselli, E. E. (1963b). The validity of management traits in relation to occupational level. *Personnel Psychology*, 16(2), pp. 109–113.
Goleman, D. (1998). *Working With Emotional Intelligence*. London: Bloomsbury.
Gottfredson, L. S. & Deary, I. J. (2004). Intelligence predicts health and longevity, but why? *Current Directions in Psychological Science*, 13(1), pp. 1–4.
Grandin, T. & Panek, R. (2014). *The Autistic Brain: Exploring the Strength of a Different Kind of Mind*. New York: First Mariner Books.

Grobman, J. (2009). A psychodynamic psychotherapy approach to the emotional problems of exceptionally and profoundly gifted adolescents and adults: a psychiatrist's experience. *Journal for the Education of the Gifted*, 33(1), pp. 106–125.

Haier, R. J. (2017). *The Neuroscience of Intelligence*. Cambridge: Cambridge University Press.

Hearst, C. (2016). *Personal Consultation Meeting*. [Skype] (Personal communication, 14 September 2016).

Horton, R. S. (2011). Parenting as a cause of narcissism: empirical support for psychodynamic and social learning theories. In: W. K. Campbell & J. D. Miller (Eds.). *Handbook of Narcissism and Narcissistic Personality Disorder*. Hoboken, NJ: John Wiley & Sons. pp. 181–190.

Hunt, E. (2011). *Human Intelligence*. New York: Cambridge University Press.

Ishak, N. M., Abidin, M. H. Z. & Bakar, A. Y. A. (2014). Dimensions of social skills and their relationship with empathy among gifted and talented students in Malaysia. *Procedia – Social and Behavioral Sciences*, 116, pp. 750–753.

ISIR. (n.d.). *The International Society for Intelligence Research*. [online] Available at: www.isir online.org/ [Accessed 18 August 2016].

Jacobsen, M.-E. (1999). *The Gifted Adult*. New York: Ballantine Books.

Jamison, K. R. (1993). *Touched with Fire*. New York: Free Press Paperbacks.

Jensen, A. R. (1998). *The G Factor: The Science of Mental Ability*. Westport, CT: Praeger Publishers.

Kanazawa, S. (2012). *The Intelligence Paradox*. Hoboken, NJ: John Wiley & Sons.

Kanigel, R. (1991). *The Man Who Knew Infinity*. London: Abacus.

Karpinski, R. I., Kinase Kolb, A. M., Tetreault, N. A. & Borowski, T. B. (2018). High intelligence: a risk factor for psychological and physiological overexcitabilities. *Intelligence*, 66, pp. 8–23.

Koestler, A. (1971). *The Act of Creation*. New York: Dell.

Kusy, M. & Holloway, E. (2009). *Toxic Workplace: Managing Toxic Personalities and Their Systems of Power*. San Francisco, CA: Jossey-Bass.

Livingston, L. A., Covert, E., Bolton, P. & Happe, F. (2018). Good social skills despite poor theory of mind: exploring compensation in autism spectrum disorder. *Journal of Child Psychology and Psychiatry*, 60(1). doi: 10.1111/jcp.12886.

Lovecky, D. V. (1986). Can you hear the flowers singing? Issues for gifted adults. *Journal of Counselling and Development*, 64, pp. 572–575.

MacCabe, J. H. (2010). *The Extremes of the Bell Curve*. Hove: Psychology Press.

Markram, K. & Markram, H. (2010). The intense world theory – A unifying theory of the neurobiology of autism. *Frontiers in Human Neuroscience*, 4, pp. 1–29.

Maupin, K. (2014). *Cheating, Dishonesty and Manipulation: Why Bright Kids Do It*. Tucson, AZ: Great Potential Press.

Meldrum, R. C., Petkovsek, M. A., Boutwell, B. B. & Young, J. T. N. (2017). Reassessing the relationship between general intelligence and self-control in childhood. *Intelligence*, 60, pp. 1–9.

Meltzer, D., Bremner, J., Hoxter, S., Wedell, D. & Wittenberg, I. (Eds.). (1975). *Explorations in Autism: A Psychoanalytical Study*. Strath Tay, Perthshire: Clunie Press.

Miller, A. (1997). *The Drama of the Gifted Child*. New York: Basic Books.

Mollon, P. (2001). *Releasing the Self – The Healing Legacy of Heiz Kohut*. London: Whurr Publishers.

Nauta, N. & Ronner, S. (2013). *Gifted Workers Hitting the Target*. Maastricht: Shaker Media.

Oleson, J. C. (2016). *Criminal Genius: A Portrait of High-IQ Offenders*. Oakland, CA: University of California Press.
Paris, J. & Phillips, J. (Eds.). (2013). *Making the DSM-5*. New York: Springer.
Persson, R. S. (2009). The unwanted gifted and talented: a sociobiological perspective of the societal functions of giftedness. In: L. V. Shavinina (Ed.). *International Handbook on Giftedness*. Quebec: Springer. pp. 913–924.
Remington, A. (2017). *The Gift of Autism*. [questions addressed following her presentation] (Personal communication, 23 February 2017).
Rhode, M. & Klauber, T. (Eds.). (2004). *The Many Faces of Asperger's Syndrome*. London: Karnac.
Robertson, K. F., Smeets, S., Lubinski, D. & Benbow, C. P. (2010). Beyond the threshold hypothesis: even among the gifted and top math/science graduate students, cognitive abilities, vocational interests, and lifestyle preferences matter for career choice, performance, and persistence. *Current Directions in Psychological Science*, 19, pp. 346–351.
Sacks, O. (2007). A bolt from the blue. *New Yorker*. 23 July 2007 issue.
Schore, A. N. (2016). *Affect Regulation and the Origin of the Self*. New York: Routledge.
Schwartz, J. A., Savolainen, J., Aaltonen, M., Merikukka, M., Paananen, R. & Gissler, M. (2015). Intelligence and criminal behavior in a total birth cohort: an examination of functional form, dimensions of intelligence, and the nature of offending. *Intelligence*, 51, pp. 108–118.
Silberman, S. (2015). *Neurotribes*. Melbourne MAM: Allen & Unwin.
Silverman, L. K. (2013). *Giftedness 101*. New York: Springer.
Simonton, D. K. (1984). *Genius, Creativity, and Leadership: Historiometric Inquiries*. London: Harvard University Press.
Simonton, D. K. (1985). Intelligence and personal influence in groups: four nonlinear models. *Psychological Review*, 92(4), pp. 532–547.
Simonton, D. K. (2009). *Genius 101*. New York: Springer.
Soanes, C., Hawker, S. & Elliott, J. (Eds.). (2006). *Paperback Oxford English Dictionary*. Oxford: Oxford University Press.
Sternberg, R. (1995). Interview with Robert Sternberg on The Bell Curve. *Skeptic*, 3(3), pp. 72–80.
Streznewski, M. K. (1999). *Gifted Grown Ups: The Mixed Blessings of Extraordinary Potential*. New York: John Wiley & Sons.
Tan, C.-M. (2012). *Search Inside Yourself*. London: HarperCollins.
The National Autistic Society Website. (n.d.). *What Is Autism?* [online] Available at: www.autism.org.uk/about/what-is/asd.aspx. [Accessed 3 May 2019].
Tustin, F. (1981). *Autistic States in Children*. (revised ed.). Reprint 1992. London: Routledge & Kegan Paul.
Tustin, F. (1990). *The Protective Shell in Children and Adults*. London: Karnac.
Vance, A. (2015). *Elon Musk*. London: Virgin Books.
Webb, J. T., Amend, E. R., Beljan, P., Webb, N. E., Kuzujanakis, M., Olenchak, F. R. & Goerss, J. (2016). *Misdiagnosis and Dual Diagnoses of Gifted Children and Adults*. (2nd ed.). Tucson, AZ: Great Potential Press.
Weismann-Arcache, C. & Tordjman, S. (2012). Relationships between depression and high intellectual potential. *Depression Research and Treatment*, 2012, pp. 1–8.
Williams, S. (2017). How 12-year old Alma Deutscher became the world's "little Mozart". *The Telegraph*. [online]. Available at: www.telegraph.co.uk/women/life/meet-prodigy-alma-deutscher-12-year-old-opera/ [Accessed 9 May 2019].

Wing, L. (1981). Asperger's Syndrome: a clinical account. *Psychological Medicine*, 11, pp. 1115–1129.

Wing, L. (1988). The continuum of autistic characteristics. In: E. Schopler & G. Mesibov (Eds.). *Diagnosis and Assessment in Autism*. New York: Plenum Press. pp. 91–110.

World Health Organization. (2018). *ICD-11: International Classification of Diseases 11th Revision*. [online] Available at: https://icd.who.int/en/ [Accessed 12 May 2019].

Wraw, C., Deary, I. J., Gale, C. R. & Der, G. (2015). Intelligence in youth and health at age 50. *Intelligence*, 53, pp. 23–32.

PART III
Implications

7
ENTRAPMENT

The unintentional perpetuation of interpersonal trouble

> **Reflective Prompt 7:** Think about an individual who you would describe as being extremely intelligent. (This could be someone you know personally, or see in the media, or it could be yourself.) Which adjectives, or nicknames, would you use – or which have you noticed others using – to describe this person? Is there any recurring pattern that you see in the role that this person tends to take up – or be assigned – in relation to others? Can you describe anything about this that you don't like? How would you like it to be different? For it to change, what do you think would be involved?

In Webb et al.'s (2016:258) chapter on "Relationships Issues for Gifted Children and Adults", they write that "Many gifted children and adults would agree that embracing their giftedness often comes with some type of social price tag". They go on to say that "Fortunately, being bright brings with it an ability to find solutions to many problems, including interpersonal ones" (Webb et al. 2016:258). However, what I noticed in my research was that interviewees' experiences of interpersonal trouble didn't always fit into the quite cognitive-sounding formula of "problems" for which they could "find solutions" – instead there could be a pervasive relational pattern that they participated in, and had become habituated to, as though that was just part of how life was for them. They seemed to experience such interpersonal patterns as something impenetrable and beyond their control, as though they were hapless victims of it. What might constitute it, or what might underlie it, was not necessarily accessible to their conscious awareness in a way that could be formulated into a problem for which a solution could be found. For example, see this excerpt, where interviewee Tracy is talking about her work colleagues:

Tracy: ... the team that I'm in now, I don't get on with my peers at all. Well it's not that I don't get on with them, but they just don't ... I'm like a complete outsider
SF: ... *So you feel they don't accept you?*
Tracy: No not at all. They don't like me.
SF: *Okay. And do you have a sense of why that is?*
Tracy: Well I've gone over it and over it really with my partner and I don't know.

I started wondering about the implications for interviewees of how they had cumulatively experienced their extreme intelligence being reacted to, and how they might have accordingly adapted themselves socially, so that they might now be unintentionally playing a part – without consciously wanting to play that part or even realising that they were – in perpetuating the troubles they were reporting. Because in all human interaction, even when a situation is experienced as though we are a passive recipient of what is happening, we are always making an active contribution to what we are experiencing (not only in our actions but also in the attitudes, expectations, and interpretations we bring to a situation). However, people in general are often not aware of how they are doing this. This chapter explores some of these unconscious processes, showing how they can help to make sense of some of the interpersonal experiences very high-IQ adults find themselves having when they do not understand why that is their experience (and why it keeps on being their experience).

The past in the present

It was Freud who pioneered an understanding of how much we are influenced by our past – particularly childhood – experiences. Extremely intelligent individuals will – like any others – also manifest long-term implications of how they have experienced being reacted to and related with. There were occasions during my research interviews when interviewees described a situation and then themselves spontaneously made an explicit link with their past, stating that it was because of what they had experienced in the past that their behaviour was the way it now was. For example Gill, who was bullied at school, is talking about avoiding participating socially at work:

> Probably the most difficult would be I worry about the office gossip ... There will be one person in particular that might be rubbing someone up the wrong way at a certain time. That sort of thing I find difficult. I worry that might become me at some point when there becomes a bit of an atmosphere, someone might walk out the room and

people start to talk and then they walk back in and everyone … it's very playground tactics really isn't it, so that I think, "Oh no, I don't want to go through all that again, I've had that at school already", so one of the reasons I keep my distance I think.

Below is another example of a present situation being interpreted in terms of what had been experienced in the past:

> And I think, you know, maybe like my previous experiences and having been bullied, I assumed that people were reacting in a negative way towards me …
>
> *(Tess)*

Tracy described not a specific incident but instead a general sense of her position in relation to others that she saw as having been set up in the past and recurring in the present:

> … it ended up meaning that I was really apart from my peers because my teachers deliberately said, "Well there's no point you doing that work because that will be too easy, so we'll set you some other work"… I can see the parallels between being at school and being at work and being apart.

The interviewees in the above examples were conscious of the way that these past experiences were being transferred into the present and affecting their present behaviour and experience. However, sometimes interviewees were not conscious of such parallels between the past and the present, and there were some such parallels that I only started to notice when closely analysing the interview transcripts. For example, there were instances where language derived from the past was transferred into the present, as with Wayne (my emphases added):

> On p. 5 of his interview transcript, he says that at school he was known "as *a smart alec*", and was not liked.
>
> Later, on p. 32, he says "I have never, ever put Mensa on an application form as one of the clubs I'm in or one of my interests, never ever put that on there, because you always look like *a smart alec* and they won't like you."

Here Wayne is not making an explicit, conscious link that his present behaviour is informed by the past, but his use of the exact same language in each situation shows that he expects that what applied in the past will apply in the present. This was also evidenced with Tracy (my emphases added):

> On p. 2 of her transcript, speaking of her childhood, she says: "My teacher was trying to get my parents involved but because my parents

were so working class, they really *worried that I was going to get ahead of myself.*"

Later, on p. 24, talking about her current workplace, she says: "But I get on well with my superiors in the sense that *so long as I don't get ahead of myself* I guess …"

In this example again an experience from the past is being transferred to the present, but not in the form of an explicit link being made consciously. It is being transferred in unconscious assumptions that the past "rules" of acceptable conduct are still what governs the present.

With other interviewees the prevalence of interpreting present situations in ways that were influenced by past formative experiences was also striking. For example, it was apparent that for Avi his predominant interpersonal preoccupation was a fear of evoking envy in others: in comparison with other interviewees his interview contained remarkably much more content relating to this theme. Here is an example:

Avi: When I was given a lot of projects there was some form of envy from my colleagues, "Hey this guy, he joined after us but he's getting a lot of projects".
SF: And what was that like for you?
Avi: It was disturbing, so I wouldn't update them on how well my projects are doing just so that they didn't know, and therefore I was expecting a reduced level of envy. But envy is very disturbing 'cos it can build walls and no, I don't like that, I feel very disturbed.

And why was it quite so disturbing for him? Compare with Harry:

Harry: If I became aware that somebody was envious of me it would make me feel very, very happy. But I'm not sure I've come across that at all.
SF: It would make you very happy?
Harry: Of course it would.
SF: Why would that make you happy do you think?
Harry: Because I've got something that the other person wishes that he had. That would make me feel nicer wouldn't it?

A clear difference between these two interviewees is that Harry had no formative experiences involving being hurt by another's envy, whereas Avi had a traumatic formative experience of being regularly beaten up by an envious father who was threatened by his young son's intelligence (see Chapter 3). Avi could be talking of his father when he says of his current boss:

… my boss sometimes is very strange in a way, that he's very encouraging as long as you don't appear as smart as him, as long as you don't talk back. But if you produce something that is way better than him – he's very good in what he's doing, the quality of work that he produces is very, very good – but if you come out with some insights that he feels threatened with, oh he comes down very hard.

These legacies from childhood are extraordinarily enduring. For example, when Gill spoke about how afraid she was of "showing herself" at work, I thought about how this related to her growing-up experiences. She had described having had no friends at primary school, wandering around the playground painfully alone. She had been at a comprehensive school where she had "a very rocky up and down time", was teased for achieving well, and felt she needed to "dumb myself down to fit in more". However, this was only one part of her early schooling experience. Later she went to a grammar school where it was "a lot easier, I felt much happier there, it did make a difference". But even though there had been other experiences since, it is that original unhappy experience that continues to colour her current adult life, making her still very sensitive to expecting she will be reacted to negatively if she freely manifests her abilities: "That's something that I think that's almost stuck with me through later life actually", she said. And there are various associated ramifications: she says that the worst thing about her at work is never saying no and then getting stressed because of having too much to do. She had said earlier that being able to help and satisfy a person's request gets a good reaction from others and makes her feel good about herself. It is as though she so much wants to avoid a repeat of the feared negative reaction from the past and is so pleased to be able to participate in an experience where it will go well with others, that she cannot decline that opportunity of having others be appreciative of her assistance, even if it is to her ultimate detriment as it ends up making her overworked and stressed.

Challenging transference

Something I find very striking in all the accounts above, is that even when interviewees described being conscious of the way their past experiences were affecting their present behaviour and experience, they were accepting this as inevitable. This meant that they went along with interpreting the present in the light of their past experience, so that their experience of current situations continued to mimic that of the past. Freud (1917) described "transference" as an experiencing of the present as though it is the same as what happened in the past, even when it might not actually be the same. To my mind the key emphasis here is that the present *might not actually be the same* as the past. The only way to intervene in the otherwise inevitable perpetuation of transference, is to cease to passively accept it. This requires making a deliberate effort to actively challenge the way a present situation is being experienced, questioning whether the way it is being experienced is accurate or whether it is a past experience that is being superimposed on the present.

As an example, we can return to Tracy's description of being baffled by why things were not going well for her interpersonally at work. After the excerpt given at the start of this chapter where she described feeling at work "like a complete outsider", she went on to say:

Tracy: (p. 31) I don't feel like I do anything wrong. I feel like I'm always trying and I'm trying not to be too much and I'm friendly, I'm nice, I try to engage people. Maybe I try too hard, maybe that's what it is, but I feel like I try with them and I don't know what else I can do really (p.32) *[Speaking of an experience during a meeting]*: ... and I can tell they're just sitting there thinking, "just shut up".

SF: (p. 33) *So why do you think they don't want to listen to you?*

Tracy: I don't know ... They either don't think that I know what I'm talking about, or that it's just spite. I don't know whether they just think, "Oh she thinks she knows everything".

SF: *Why would they want to be spiteful towards you?*

Tracy: I don't know if they are threatened by me or ... there's definite bad feeling and I don't really know what it's from, I really don't. I've thought about it a lot.

SF: *... So to the best of your ability you are really trying to go down well with the team as much as you can, but there's something that's a bit of a mystery about quite why it's not happening?*

Tracy: Yeah, and I can only think that it's because they think that I'm a clever clogs, a know-it-all or something.

Here she is saying that she does not know why things are difficult with these colleagues, given that she is consciously doing (or at least saying that she is doing) all she possibly can to try to make things go well and yet they are not improving. Why might this be – is she right that they are simply prejudiced against her because she is clever?

A first step in trying to make sense of this is to challenge whether the way the current situation is being experienced is accurate, or whether it is a passive perpetuation of transference. During Tracy's childhood she experienced herself as being very different from her family of origin – perhaps "like a complete outsider". For example, she described that "my parents aren't the sort of people to sit down with a book and read to their child", whereas "I always had my nose in a book", and "nothing's changed". She was IQ tested at school and based on the results was offered a place at a prestigious grammar school, but her parents would not let her go there. This made her very resentful towards them:

> I moved out of my dad's house when I was 17 and started living on my own. I'd just turned 17. I'd had a big row with him and left home.
> Suffice to say I don't have a brilliant relationship with my parents now. They really didn't want me to excel in that way.

I wondered how much Tracy might have been transferring onto her workplace group what she had experienced in her family group, so that she was in the present perceiving herself as different from the group, and them being hostile towards her and not wanting her to excel, just as had been the case in the past. Speaking again of her workplace:

> As long as I just stood by the photocopier and did ... she really didn't like the fact that I'd been almost promoted from under her nose, and that I wasn't under her command anymore, and I got the intense feeling ... she was very nice to me when I left, which surprised me, she was a bit odd like that, but it was clear that she didn't like that. It was like she felt that I was a bit big for my boots if you know what I mean ...

Did this person actually feel that way about her? Tracy was surprised when "she was very nice to me when I left". Of course she could be right that these staff were resentful of her progress, and maybe this co-worker was being nice to her precisely because of being pleased she was leaving. However, Tracy has said that the reason she thinks this colleague disliked her is that "I was a bit big for my boots": this is a clear legacy from her childhood, where she was given the message that she was not to "get ahead of myself". Tracy is seeing that dynamic everywhere, interpreting others' reactions in terms of this formative experience, assuming they are the same, when perhaps in current situations others might not actually mind her excelling in the same way that her family minded when she was growing up.

At one point in her interview Tracy said "My peers I would think, see maybe it's all just in my head, but my peers I would think they would say I'm overbearing ...". Here she is starting to suggest that perhaps there could be a different way of interpreting her current experience – "maybe it's all just in my head". Being willing to challenge one's default interpretation of a situation is one way to begin to dispense with old patterns.

A second step in making sense of baffling interpersonal experiences, is to become more aware of one's own, sometimes quite subtle, attitudes and behaviours that influence interactions. For example, talking about her older sister, Tracy said:

> That was a difficult relationship growing up. Can you imagine being three years older and your little kid sister's a lot cleverer than you? There was a lot of jealousy on her part from when we were growing up, definitely. I can't blame her really, I probably didn't do anything to help the situation ... That must have been really difficult for her.

Here she is acknowledging that in this relationship in the past, she herself played a part in fuelling the interpersonal difficulties: "I probably didn't do anything to help the situation".

148 Implications

Having developed (in relation to her sister) an identity of being "the cleverer one", gave Tracy recognition for something important about herself – her intellectual ability – and also affirmed her power to compete successfully. Sibling rivalry is for most of us our first experience of grappling with competition. Gaining an identity as "the cleverer one" is something that Tracy can therefore be expected to have taken some delight in and to have wanted to perpetuate, even though it came with difficulties such as jealousy and family conflict.

I wondered whether these experiences might have left Tracy with an equation that being clever means being resented by others, so that relinquishing interpersonal difficulty could feel like relinquishing her intellectual ability. If in her current life she is still invested in perpetuating this identity of being "the cleverer one", it might involve continuing to fuel others' resentment just as she did with her sister, because this identity, together with the interpersonal difficulty it brings, is her familiar way of feeling validated by others.

Valency

To revisit, with a different emphasis, something that we looked at before, recall how Tracy described that when she started a new job she was treated:

> ... like I was the messiah ... because every meeting that I went into, they were just like, "Oh god we've been waiting for somebody like you [Tracy], we're so happy".

We can analyse how Tracy might be invested in seeing things this way and in behaving in ways that facilitate such reactions from others. However, this is never just about one individual's behaviour – whatever happens is always a combination of ongoing recognition and interaction that is occurring between the individual and the environment (see Chapter 3). The above excerpt portrays these members of staff as clearly wanting, and waiting for, a messiah. People do seek someone who they can look up to, be impressed by, trust, be led by, mimicking the infant's seeking of a safety-inducing experience with a strong and reliable caregiver. The longing for such a leader is evident in the popularity of many religions that identify a powerful figure who one is enjoined to fully trust and submit to. This is not always positive – it is also how fascist dictators and toxic CEOs are enabled to secure and retain their reigns. Submitting to a leader, whether a supernaturally conceived one or a mortal human one, is – as Gimbernat (2013) has argued – a primitive instinct that has served an important evolutionary purpose. There are better prospects of survival for individuals who group together, and such groups function more coherently when co-operating in accordance with a sanctioned leadership. A person who demonstrates impressively capable performance and persuasively articulated strategic vision can start to assume the position of leader, both because of his or her own commanding behaviour, but also because of the propensity for submission that others, in the face of such behaviour, yield to.

A useful way of conceptualising this is provided by the Systemic concept of "valency". This term derives from chemistry, referring to how the properties of an atom give it the power to combine with certain other atoms in specific ways that form particular compounds. Bion (1961) first adapted this concept to apply it to people's behaviour in groups, using it to signify what propensity a person has for getting into which kinds of social dynamics with other people. Valency is a readiness (unconscious) to take up a certain position in relation to others that triggers matching responses from those others, causing a familiar compound of interpersonal dynamics to recur albeit in new contexts and with different individuals. Extremely intelligent individuals have a valency for taking up certain typical positions in relation to others – such as Tracy's position of "messiah", or interviewee Erik's position of "an oracle" (see Chapter 3). Those around them participate in assigning to extremely intelligent individuals certain typical social roles or functions, such as those Persson (2009) identified as "the nerd", "the hero", and "the martyr". The way interpersonal experiences unfold between a high-IQ individual and others is therefore never solely about the conscious control that any one person alone can exert, as it always includes the dynamic interaction of various systemic elements.

Repetition compulsion

Even where one person can exert control over an aspect of their lives that is unsatisfying, they may not do so. Coined by Freud (1920), "repetition compulsion" refers to how we can adhere repetitively to preserving the way things were in the past, even if how they were was negative. For example, interviewee Wayne described (in Chapter 4) how he did not fit in at school, where he "messed around" and "misbehaved". He said that in his current life (just as was the case at school), his intelligence was "totally under-used". He expressed bitterness that something was not made of him, provided for him, at a young age, that he was not nurtured more, that he was not in a more testing environment where he could have achieved more. He told how his parents did not show pride in his abilities, and he had no career guidance at school. After school he went to work in a factory. He said that he used to live at home and go out with friends and "just generally waste time and waste life I think". It appeared he was trying to keep out of the house, as he said when he was home his dad was quite authoritarian, and "If I'm not in the way, I'm not a problem". He said he had a general feeling that "things have conspired against me". These distressing lacks he experienced appear to sensitise him to distress elsewhere: he described feeling the problems of the world acutely – "You realise how much really is wrong with the world, and when you read a newspaper about a child dying from neglect or abuse it really, really hurts now". It is as though he sees in this, himself as the neglected child, with the high potential that was identified in him having died. "It's the one thing", he said, "that brings me close to tears".

Even though Wayne expressed significant distress at his past experience of being neglected, something that comes across in his narrative is his passivity in accepting the dissatisfaction of his present life. He likens his current experience to that of the past but leaves it at that, when the possibility exists of playing an active part in making the present different from the past. In this respect, it seems there is almost a compulsion to repeat the earlier experiences. He had described how his parents did not do enough for him while growing up, yet it could be said that he is repeating this by not doing enough for himself now. It is as though he is still waiting for someone else to come forward as the better parent and redeem the neglect.

Another example is that, just as he said he felt different from others growing up and did not fit in, he described that now, even at Mensa, he is different, he is not like other Mensa members – "They would smile at me, they would talk to me, but they wouldn't like me". Here he is insisting that however convivially people behave towards him now, they still do not like him, just as was the case in the past. One component underlying this repetition could be that once you have become familiar with experiencing yourself as different and not fitting in, being different can become part of your identity so that it becomes uncomfortable to think you could belong with or be like others. You might then come to (unconsciously) preserve that self-concept of being different from others, selectively non-attending to the ways in which you might be similar to others. Because there are lots of basic ways in which all of us are similar to each other if it is similarity that is being sought.

Comparably, although Tracy spoke of having had a tough background and not receiving the support or help she needed, she now in some ways perpetuates this situation. During the interview I asked whether she thought it would be useful if there was more understanding around the issues that high-IQ people face:

SF: *Do you think … it would be in some way useful to somebody like you if in society there was a way of thinking about that [extreme intelligence] differently, or people understanding it differently?*

Tracy: I think in some sense possibly. However it is a gift and it is an advantage, I suppose, depending on your point of view, and so to try to help bring people in to give them more of an advantage seems a bit wrong if you like. To try and get them a level playing field, I suppose, because you would hope that people who are gifted would rise to the top in whatever field naturally, organically, so do you need that additional understanding?

It is clear that she has not herself "rise[n] to the top … naturally", she has worked very hard and struggled significantly for many years – "It sounds like [my life's] this big tragic story in many ways of lack of love and all of that" – yet she says it "seems a bit wrong" to consider changing things. It is as though she is seeking to preserve the situation that involves herself and others like her not being understood. She does not seem to want to change her familiar view of very high IQ as something that you do not get support for, you have to tough it out and find your own way to something better, against various people's hostility and resentment, alone.

Change, and resistance to change

Intellectual giftedness has, as Yermish (2010) puts it, a pervasive influence on the self. High-IQ attributes, intertwined with how these have been interpersonally responded to, become a strong part of a person's identity. (Recall in Chapter 3 how important interviewees rated their high IQ as being in their personal identity.) Just as much as any person might derive a sense of security from relying on a sense of identity of some kind, and engage in defending it against perceived threats of denigration or disintegration, so too will high-IQ individuals protect the foundations of their particular identity. If their identity has been built through being set apart from others, then however uncomfortable being set apart might have been for them, it becomes the familiar position, the kind of familiar life position that Berne (1961) maintains we use our social interactions to try to affirm. High-IQ individuals might therefore keep endorsing themselves as being different from others (as Wayne did) because this distinctness forms their familiar self-image and therefore underpins their self-esteem. In this way they might become involved in perpetuating that identity regardless of its social drawbacks.

Given that, as we have seen in Chapter 3, a person has an inbuilt drive to seek recognition, it appears that the extremely intelligent person continues to try to seek recognition even if the way they go about this provokes others, because getting a reaction of some kind is preferable to being ignored. When a person has become habituated to a negative reaction – as had Tracy – they could continue to unconsciously play their part in eliciting a negative reaction because it is at least a way of having this important aspect of their identity in some way interpersonally engaged with. Berne (1961) asserts that we need acknowledgement from others – what he terms "strokes" – whether this is positive or negative. He maintains that a negative stroke is preferable to no stroke.

Once a person has established a view of themselves and others and of what to expect of others and therefore how to relate with others, this map (or internal working model) becomes the known, the familiar. Even if this is negative, limiting, and causes isolation and distress, it is a distress that is familiar and has already been adapted to. Remaining trapped in this can therefore be less anxiety-provoking than having to forge a new, unknown way which might prove demanding and perhaps (it is feared) be ultimately disappointing or even worse than the prevailing status quo. Psychodynamic theory explains that we resist something – such as a change –

when we anticipate it could cause anxiety and pain. By resisting change we are attempting to defend ourselves against anxiety and pain.

Paradoxically, however, it is also true that even the envisaging of a change that could be perceived to be a change for the better can in itself bring pain – what Casement calls "the pain of contrast" (1990:106). This is the painfulness of realising just how difficult things have been, as occasioned by encountering the contrast between the familiar difficult situation and the possibilities of a better situation that are beginning to be apprehended. This pain can be defended against by aborting the process of proceeding with something that is potentially better, thereby rejecting any change. By sticking with a view that the difficulty of things is, or has been, inevitable, what is avoided is an experiencing of the acute pain of regret or resentment that could come with accepting that things could have been better, that easier is possible. This can also fuel a resistance to making things easier for others, thereby avoiding the pain of feeling envy towards others who might be afforded the advantage of an easier time than you yourself have had. This appears relevant to Tracy when she resisted the suggestion of promoting better understanding and support for individuals with high IQ.

The point, however, in going through the kind of detailed analysis presented above is that it can be helpful for someone to realise that they are playing a part in perpetuating the troubles they are experiencing. Realising that one might unconsciously be actively contributing to an unwanted situation can be liberating because it introduces the option of identifying what one's part in this is and then making a deliberate choice and effort to change the related attitudes, expectations, interpretations, and actions. Identifying these components can be hard, and changing them even harder, because it entails breaking through the pain barrier (pain of change) and then with regular repetition instating new habits. However, if there is the appetite for it then it is a project that can be actively embraced with the possibility of significant rewards to be gained, as opposed to simply continuing passively with an unhappy and confounding status quo.

Summary

It is apparent from this chapter that when extremely high-IQ individuals experience interpersonal difficulty in their lives, sometimes it can be that they are implicated in perpetuating it in ways that they might not be aware of. It is when individuals find themselves participating in dynamics that they are baffled by that the concept of unconscious processes can be helpful in elucidating what might be going on. This chapter has engaged with the Psychodynamic concepts of transference and repetition compulsion (Freud) and the Systemic concept of valency (Bion).

The chapter has emphasised – to paraphrase the slogan seen on posters around London advertising Mark Ravenhill's play "The Cane" – that the past never stays where you think you left it. It has been shown how extraordinarily enduring the effects can be of formative social experiences. It has also been shown that even if the recurring interpersonal patterns that these create are distressing, and a person realises this and is offered a way out, he or she might resist change, avoiding the effort, fear of the unknown, and "pain of contrast" (Casement) involved. It has been highlighted that the rationale for becoming aware of these unconscious processes, challenging them and pushing through the pain barrier to make a change, is that one can thereby become liberated from the constrictions of dissatisfying old habits and patterns. To achieve change it is also necessary to become aware of how systems tend to assign certain typical roles to those who manifest extreme intelligence, and to notice and challenge the way that different individuals within a system play their parts in this with related behaviours and expectations.

References

Berne, E. (1961). *Transactional Analysis in Psychotherapy: A Systematic Individual and Social Psychiatry*. New York: Grove Press.

Bion, W. (1961). *Learning from Experience*. London: Heinemann Medical Books.

Casement, P. (1990). *Further Learning from the Patient*. London: Routledge.

Freud, S. (1917). Transference. In: J. Strachey (Ed.). *The Standard Edition of the Complete Psychological Works of Sigmund Freud Volume 1*. Reprint 1991. London: Penguin Books. pp. 482–500.

Freud, S. (1920). Beyond the pleasure principle. In: J. Strachey (Ed.). *The Standard Edition of the Complete Psychological Works of Sigmund Freud Volume XVIII*. Reprint 2001. London: Vintage, pp. 7–65.

Gimbernat, A. (2013). *The Lust for Reverence*. Mechanicsburg, PA: Sunbury Press.

Persson, R. S. (2009). The unwanted gifted and talented: a sociobiological perspective of the societal functions of giftedness. In: L. V. Shavinina (Ed.). *International Handbook on Giftedness*. Quebec: Springer. pp. 913–924.

Webb, J. T., Amend, E. R., Beljan, P., Webb, N. E., Kuzujanakis, M., Olenchak, F. R. & Goerss, J. (2016). *Misdiagnosis and Dual Diagnoses of Gifted Children and Adults*. (2nd ed.). Tucson, AZ: Great Potential Press.

Yermish, A. (2010). *Cheetahs on the Couch: Issues Affecting the Therapeutic Working Alliance with Clients Who are Cognitively Gifted*. Unpublished PhD thesis, Massachusetts School of Professional Psychology.

8

HIDING SELF, REACHING OUT

The "High-IQ Relational Styles" framework

> **Reflective Prompt 8:** Many frameworks have been created for trying to make sense of people's interpersonal feelings and behaviours – for example Myers-Briggs, the Big Five, the Enneagram, even Zodiac Signs and Chinese Horoscopes. When you think of yourself and others, do you make use of any such framework? Which one? What do you find useful about such a framework? What are its limitations? What do you know about how the framework was derived?

Numerous representations of interpersonal relating in extremely intelligent individuals have been provided in the preceding chapters. The current chapter draws all of this together and sets out an original conceptual framework which I have created to depict the central styles of interaction that I have discerned through analysing my research interviews and professional practice with very high-IQ individuals, as well as my textual analysis of literature and research on giftedness and high IQ. This four-quadrant framework – titled "High-IQ Relational Styles" – shows how these styles relate to one another, and to the Naive Child and Arrogant Emperor profiles introduced in Chapter 5. The first sections of the current chapter explain each of the four quadrants of the framework one by one, making reference to relevant examples. The final sections discuss the framework as a whole, comparing it with the work of several giftedness authors as well as showing how it relates to several established mainstream psychological theories on interpersonal relating. The Appendix at the end of the book provides more detail about how I derived this framework from my research data.

Introducing and explaining the framework

My framework does not categorise types of people, but styles of interpersonal relating. Different people might fall predominantly into one or other of these styles of relating, but the same person could at different times (for example different periods of his or her life) or in different contexts, relate in predominantly one or other of these ways. It can also be viewed as different parts within a person's own interpersonal repertoire or potential repertoire, so that a person can move between quadrants in different situations, or their predominant style of relating can show growth from one quadrant to another or regression back from one to another.

The framework distils two main dimensions of interpersonal relating: expressiveness of self, and acceptance by others. The "expressiveness of self" dimension links with the "Person" element of the High-IQ Context model (Chapter 3), in that an extremely high-IQ person has certain distinctive attributes and has different options available to him- or herself for whether or how to express these, from low expressiveness through to high expressiveness. The "acceptance by others" dimension links with the "Environment" element of the High-IQ Context model, as it relates to the environmental response received. How much acceptance a high-IQ person's expressiveness of his or her self meets with, from low acceptance through to high acceptance, can differ in different kinds of environment, as shown in preceding chapters. Figure 8.1 represents the framework graphically, which is followed by a written explication.

If two lines are drawn – one horizontal, one vertical – that intersect in the middle, each line representing the continuum of one of the described

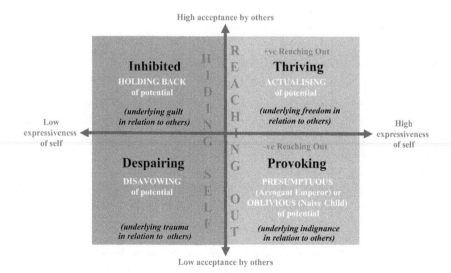

FIGURE 8.1 High-IQ Relational Styles framework

dimensions (expressiveness of self, acceptance by others) from low to high, this creates four quadrants. For each quadrant I have proposed a dominant way of being interpersonally (in large black lettering), a dominant way of relating to one's abilities or potential (in white lettering), and in black italics a dominant underlying issue that fuels the way of being interpersonally but which is often outside of the person's conscious awareness. The framework associates style of interpersonal relating (the large black lettering) with the actualising of high-IQ potential (the white lettering). This association between interpersonal relating and the actualising of potential is well-established in the literature (Towers 1987, Jacobsen 1999; Streznewski 1999; Nauta & Corten 2002; Persson 2009) and is further elaborated later in this chapter where the High-IQ Relational Styles framework is linked with the work of other authors.

The two quadrants shaded dark grey on the left-hand side depict lower levels of expressiveness of self, which I have labelled "Hiding Self", whilst the two quadrants shaded lighter grey on the right-hand side depict higher levels of expressiveness, which I have labelled "Reaching Out". Reaching Out can be undertaken in a way that is positive (top right quadrant) or negative (bottom right quadrant).

Hiding Self

The way that extremely intelligent individuals might resort to hiding themselves has been introduced at the end of Chapter 4 and referred to again towards the end of Chapter 5. Here a deeper analysis of this phenomenon is provided, showing how it can develop in different versions which I have termed "Inhibited" or "Despairing".

Top left quadrant: Inhibited

If someone has on the whole experienced acceptance from others, yet still chooses to hide themselves, i.e. to limit their expressiveness of their abilities, what is going on? Based on my research interviews and textual analysis of relevant literature, I hypothesise that a person in such a state is holding themselves back out of concern that in fully expressing themselves, they might harm others. This is the inhibition that by expressing yourself freely, what is good about you could cause others to feel bad about themselves. It is an inhibition about being "too big", "too much" (such as my interviewee John expressed), and that by taking up positions yourself you are preventing others from holding those positions and therefore could cause disappointment or distress to others or retribution (such as interviewee Tracy expressed in connection with feeling disliked for having been promoted at work). Also included here is feeling sorry for others when it is noticed that others might try really hard but not manage to achieve something you have been able to achieve (and which you may have achieved without having had to try very hard, as was expressed by interviewees Mei and Erik). It is an uncomfortable feeling that – and this is an inevitability in any competitive situation – your success is built on others' failure: you have become the winner only by someone else having become the loser (as Tracy alluded to when she spoke of her team being slimmed down at work, and how it was expected that she would be kept on whilst others would lose their jobs). This kind of experience can leave high-IQ individuals feeling guilty about their abilities, with a wish to hold themselves back: they hide themselves so as to protect the well-being of others and to protect themselves from negative reactions. For example interviewee Gill:

> I have felt like it must be difficult for other people, and that is another thing that makes me hold back on it because I don't want to make people feel even worse if they are feeling bad about it.

Also with interviewee John, there was a strong family message that he and his siblings were each to keep away from participating seriously in any activity that one of the others had already shown an interest in. This rooted out competitiveness, preventing it from being seen as something that could be healthy and even enjoyable and engaged in with robustness. This left John, as the youngest of four siblings, with an imperative not to displace anyone else by himself succeeding. He has ever since applied his considerable abilities in various directions but stopped short of reaching the top, deferring to someone else (perhaps representing an older sibling) in relation to whom he chooses to take up second position. The top left quadrant represents this situation: a person has not been hindered by lack of acceptance from others, but holds themselves back out of an underlying guilt in relation to others which they may or may not be consciously aware of. They are concerned that by fully expressing and actualising their own potential they could cause harm to others, and they want to prevent this from happening.

The thinking in this quadrant is particularly supported by Grobman's work (2006; 2009). He describes working with gifted clients who – even though as children they were generally admired and popular and rarely subjected to malicious envy – evinced an irrational belief that succeeding in using their powerful intellect would humiliate others. He found that they felt ashamed, embarrassed, and guilty about their abilities, and quietly tried to figure out ways to equalise the differences that had become apparent between themselves and their peers. For these individuals, it was not a poor environmental fit but rather their unconscious ways of trying to hide their potential that caused problems. Freeman (2010:29) also writes about gifted individuals hiding themselves, and the phenomenon of gifted people themselves setting up internal barriers (Freeman 2010:191) rather than it being others who are obstructing them.

Bottom left quadrant: Despairing

If someone has had such low acceptance from others that it qualifies as neglect or abuse, and the person has been traumatised by this, they could completely shut down on expressing themselves, disavowing their potential out of a despair that there is no point. Interviewees who had traumatic experience included Avi and John, who were regularly beaten by their fathers for being strong-willed and questioning. How a person is affected by such experiences can change over time and according to what other influences they experience. So, for example, at my time of studying John's predominant way of relating, in spite of his earlier trauma I saw him – as described in the previous section – as being "Inhibited", not "Despairing". As an adult John had had a lot of therapy, which will have influenced the effects on him of the trauma he had experienced early in life. The situation depicted in the bottom left "Despairing" quadrant is one in which a high-IQ person is – at that point in time – giving up, dropping out. This was evident in interviewee Wayne's narrative of himself as a somewhat neglected child who as an adult had given up on trying to find ways to employ his high intelligence, and who suffered from depression. Tracy described a period of her life during which she was "in a self-imposed exile", "very closed off". Helene talked of having experienced being "badly depressed and feeling on the verge of suicidal tendencies". Such experience was also evident in a high-IQ client of mine who aborted her pregnancy out of despair that there could be a good place in the world for her foetus with whom she said she felt she had already fallen in love: she wanted to rescue it from a life as difficult as she had found her own to be. Another example is interviewee Bonnie, who experienced school as being so pointless that she truanted extensively then dropped out, turning to crime, which resulted in her spending four years in prison. In this quadrant the dominant way of being interpersonally is despairing. In these cases the underlying issue is trauma in relation to others. Such trauma can be caused by violence or abuse, but also by experiences of such misattunement, disappointment, or neglect that there is a loss of faith in others as interested, reliable, respect-worthy, or relevant. This can bring about a losing of hope in making any attempt to express the deeper or more unique aspects of yourself, because – based on what you have experienced so far – you have no reason to expect that expressing yourself could be effectively responded to. A fear could also be harboured that expressing yourself could make things worse by triggering rejection, violence, abandonment.

Experiencing interpersonal trauma can lead to a disavowal of high ability. Cross et al. (1993) document the coping strategies that gifted adolescents use of burying their abilities in order to avoid the stigmatisation they experience their giftedness as attracting. This also relates to Fiedler's (2015) depiction of "the invisible ones", who are gifted individuals who have disavowed engaging in any way with their potential. Yermish (2010:42) describes the ordinary, non-specialised schooling that gifted individuals are often subjected to, as delivering a series of "microaggressions" that can amount to the gifted individual becoming traumatised. Favier-Townsend (2014) described this situation as involving "intellectual neglect", leading to low self-esteem, underachievement, and lifelong regret. The bullying that extremely intelligent individuals frequently experience in school, as mentioned by several of my interviewees and documented in the literature (Peterson & Ray 2006a; 2006b), is something that can have extremely negative long-term effects into adulthood: a study by Lereya et al. (2015) shows that bullying by peers can produce more long-term anxiety, depression, and self-harm than maltreatment of children by adults, including their parents.

Reaching Out

Where an extremely intelligent person is not hiding themselves but instead is in their interpersonal behaviour reaching out to others, this can be done in a negative way – which I have termed "Provoking" – or in a positive way, which I have termed "Thriving".

Bottom right quadrant: Provoking

Where a person has expressed themselves and experienced low acceptance but of a kind that has not been severe enough to be traumatic, they might engage in increasingly exaggerating their expressing of themselves as a way of trying to gain more acceptance. This is depicted in the bottom right-hand side quadrant. This behaviour can be true of the Arrogant Emperor and also of the Naive Child – albeit for different reasons – because both of these involve experiencing a lack of receiving a satisfying response from others. The Emperor is presumptuous of his potential, expecting that he is entitled to certain attendant rewards or privileges, and is disappointed, angry, aggrieved, and arrogantly accusing of others that he is not receiving the acknowledgment he feels he deserves. With the Child, she is oblivious of her potential, but is annoyed, hurt, distressed, and disturbed that others are not understanding her, that she is naively causing inexplicable negative reactions in them. In such interaction, you are reaching out to others, but you can be doing so in a negative way because the low acceptance you have received can create in you a dominant underlying indignation in relation to others, and so the way you express yourself can be provoking of others and therefore unlikely to gain higher levels of acceptance. Such behaviour is adversarial: when a person interacts with naivety or arrogance, others are likely to withdraw or retaliate, shutting out any opportunities to form alliances and collaborate. As a person becomes more and more driven by their own sense of indignation at not receiving the response they hope for, they can become less and less in touch with what is driving the reactions of others. The kind of interpersonal difficulty that results has been shown in Chapter 5. The following interview extract gives an example of this sort of interaction, in which the high-IQ individual might not be aware of the indignance that underlies her way of relating to someone, and how that is causing a negative response in the other ("getting his back up"). In talking about it, this interviewee (Helene) started becoming more aware of how she was provoking the other:

Helene: Even my [music] teacher. We butt heads regularly, because he's used to people who will take his word as gospel.
SF: Okay.
Helene: And every time I come into the studio, if I don't understand, if I don't agree, I'm going to say so. Well I'm there to learn. I'm not going to learn unless I ask the questions, but he finds that really difficult at times. The last lesson of this year was a total disaster, because he was getting his back up and I was being perfectly pleasant and just asking questions.
SF: Or so you thought?
Helene: Or so I thought, yes. Exactly. Oh dear. I was being stubborn.

In this situation, Helene starts out portraying herself as innocently "just asking questions", but rather than her questions indeed being "perfectly pleasant", or even neutral, it is as though they are fuelled by an indignance accumulated over her many years (particularly during her formative school years, as she described in her interview) of experiencing her questions not being well-received or answered, so that the way she now asks questions is already pre-loaded with what is almost an accusation of the other's anticipated inadequacy at responding satisfactorily.

An extreme example of relating that falls into this quadrant is a high-IQ client of mine who explained that she quite deliberately developed anorexia to provoke those around her. This was a kind of angry protest against others plus a desperate attempt to get some kind of attention that she was lacking. The more "out of sync" with others such reaching out to others is, the less acceptance is elicited, and the more indignant this can aggravate the person to become. In such a situation, the benign hostility (or even less than benign) that they receive from others becomes a familiar reaction and in the absence of something more rewarding, that familiar level of hostility itself becomes addictive as a kind of negative affirmation of themselves and they will seek that kind of relating rather than no relating (recalling Berne's (1961) assertion that receiving a negative stroke is better than no stroke). The underlying issue fuelling the way that individuals in this state relate with others, therefore, is their indignance in relation to others for not giving them the positive affirmation they are seeking, and which they continue to seek but with ill-judged or misguided efforts.

Freeman (2010:28) writes about the "ongoing anger" that gifted individuals can be left with when they have continually experienced environments that do not cater to their special needs. Corten et al. (2006) state that gifted individuals can become so used to not fitting in, that "by sometimes stating their opinions too categorically, they provoke their own exclusion". This describes a situation where the person is not feeling inhibited and holding back out of guilt, nor disavowing their abilities in despair because of being traumatised. Rather, they are expressing themselves fully but in a way that provokes lack of acceptance, even rejection.

Top right quadrant: Thriving

The top right quadrant depicts interpersonal relating that is characterised by a person's high expressiveness of self together with experiencing high levels of acceptance by others. An example of someone living in this state is interviewee Hugh. He has a satisfying and valued 22-year-long relationship with his partner, and has specifically maintained contact with all the friends he has made throughout his life except one. Professionally, he is applying a sophistication of interpersonal skill to the effective navigating of a wide range of roles, at a very senior level, with a balance between expressing himself incisively but doing so in a way that is always monitoring others' needs and feelings. He is very patient about choosing the best timing for expressing himself. This kind of careful judgment brings about in return an experiencing of positive feedback and high levels of professional, personal, and material success. In his dealings with others, there is noticeably a distinct lack of either naivety or arrogance. There is also a full engagement with both competition and collaboration, but from the "safe" position of having established a secure base. This can also impart a sense of safety to others: enough others are experiencing Hugh as an ally, rather than an adversary, so that he is being offered many opportunities for collaboration with others. This combination brings about a predominant way of being interpersonally that comprises thriving. In this state, a high-IQ person is able to actualise their potential as they are fully expressing themselves, but they are doing so in a way that is "in sync" with others and which therefore generates high acceptance by others. A person in such a state is reaching out to others in a positive rather than a negative way. Based on cultivating an openness to feedback from others, and continually working to improve your interpersonal understanding and skill, you can evolve your way of expressing yourself. This results in increasing your effectiveness at communication, rather than provoking others or resorting to hiding yourself. In this situation the underlying issue fuelling interpersonal relating is a freedom in relation to others: there is nothing restricting your relating with others, skewing it in a particular direction. This is not to say that a person in such a state is greeted with acceptance by everyone in every situation all of the time, but the overall interpersonal picture is as described.

Examples of such interpersonal thriving and actualising of potential are provided by Towers (1987) in his description of gifted individuals who become "pillars of the community", and in Streznewski's (1999) description of "superstars" who are outstanding in the way that they are both noticeably excelling in their chosen activities and occupations and are noticeably connected with others and happy.

Moving between quadrants

The High-IQ Relational Styles framework allows for people's ways of functioning to be changeable and shift rather than remain static. Within the framework, optimal functioning is what is encapsulated in the "Thriving" quadrant. In other words, looking at that top-right "Thriving" quadrant in Figure 8.1, optimal functioning is seen as functioning that is fuelled by an underlying sense of freedom in relation to others (the black italics), involving a person predominantly reaching out to others in a positive rather than negative way (the grey lettering), and in which a person is able to actualise their potential (the white lettering). The ideal process of development for any person, therefore, would be to increasingly be able to function in the way that is represented in that top-right "Thriving" quadrant. This means that, if the way that a person predominantly functions can be situated in one of the two dark-grey-shaded left-hand side "Hiding Self" quadrants or in the bottom right-hand side "negative Reaching Out" quadrant, then making a shift from any of those three quadrants' ways of functioning towards a way of functioning that involves a "positive Reaching Out" (top-right quadrant) would be seen as worthwhile development. Another way of describing this, is by referring to the layer of how a person relates to their abilities or potential (the white lettering). Ways of functioning that involve predominantly "Holding Back" (top-left quadrant) high-IQ potential, or "Disavowing" (bottom-left quadrant) such potential, or being "Presumptuous" or "Oblivious" (bottom-right quadrant) of their potential, are all ways of functioning that do not facilitate a fulfilling of potential. Making a shift, therefore, towards a way of functioning that involves "Actualising" that potential (top-right quadrant), would be seen as a worthwhile process of development. How movement can take place towards that top-right "Thriving" quadrant from any of the other three quadrants is addressed in the next chapter (Chapter 9, "Helping high ability thrive").

Movement within the framework can also take place in other directions. For example, a person whose relational style is predominantly "Provoking" (bottom-right quadrant) could over time experience such negative reactions from others that cumulatively this becomes traumatising, and they begin to move into a predominantly "Despairing" way of functioning (bottom-left quadrant, where there is an underlying sense of trauma in relation to others). A person whose way of functioning is situated in the top-right "Thriving" quadrant can also move backwards (i.e. leftwards to a quadrant at the left-hand side of Figure 8.1) or downwards (to a quadrant at the bottom of Figure 8.1). An example is a client of mine who enjoyed an early childhood during which family acceptance engendered in her a sense of freedom in expressing herself in relation to others. Her predominant relational style of "Thriving" came to be significantly challenged, however, when she started attending an ill-matching school. There – as unfortunately so often happens to extremely high-IQ individuals in unsuitable environments – she began to feel uncomfortable about who and what she was in relation to what she was seeing of others around her and how they were responding to her, which caused a "Holding Back" of herself to begin to develop, moving her into the "Inhibited" quadrant (top left-hand side quadrant in Figure 8.1). In this kind of situation of changed circumstances it could also be that a person who was "Thriving" comes to react to a loss of satisfying responsiveness from others by becoming "Provoking" (bottom right-hand side quadrant), reaching out in a negative way towards others by being accusatory or critical towards them and trying to demand a more satisfying response. Equally, becoming interpersonally traumatised could cause a person who was once "Thriving" to move into "Despairing" (bottom-left quadrant).

Linking High-IQ Relational Styles with other giftedness life-strategies/trajectories

Several authors (Towers 1987, Jacobsen 1999; Streznewski 1999; Nauta & Corten 2002; Persson 2009) have identified different categories of life-strategy or trajectory that are noticeable within a high-IQ/gifted population, but none of these authors relate their work to each other's or to mainstream psychological theories. One author who has related her work to mainstream psychological theories is Fiedler (2012; 2015), who looks at the development of gifted adults across the lifespan and maps this onto Erikson's (1950) psychosocial stages of development. She is not categorising different overall life-strategies or trajectories, however, but looking at the challenges associated with particular age ranges from age 18 onwards and ways of handling such challenges. All of these authors comment on how gifted individuals relate to others and how they actualise their potential, and they all present these two issues as being highly interrelated. Each author emphasises a slightly different angle, for example socioeconomic background (Towers 1987), attitude to life (Jacobsen 1999), individual career performance (Nauta & Corten 2002), or function in society (Persson 2009).

Table 8.1 shows how the categories put forward by each of these authors relate to each other, and to the different quadrants of my High-IQ Relational Styles framework. A summary of these authors' categories follows.

Towers (1987) identifies three different kinds of adjustment, based on the type of childhood experienced and its socioeconomic environment. The first, he calls the "committed strategy". Here, an individual grows up in an upper middle-class environment, with parents who are gifted and well-educated, attends prestigious colleges and enters matching occupations, and has friends with similar histories. Towers asserts that these are the gifted individuals who are optimally adjusted, who are "pillars of the community". Those with a "marginal strategy" grow up in a lower socioeconomic class, may not even have gone to college, and take on perhaps menial jobs but in their own time pursue their original and less mainstream interests. He describes his third category – "dropouts" – as possibly having gifted parents but who themselves are maladjusted, who use the child to try to fulfil their own ambitions and gratify their own needs for accomplishment.

TABLE 8.1 High-IQ Relational Styles and other authors' giftedness life-strategies/trajectories

Author	Excelling, outstandingly successful	Doing well, works hard, adapting	Original, but difficult to deal with, not collaborating	Not demonstrating, or not being appreciated for, the value they can offer	Dropping out
Towers (1987)	Committed strategy		Marginal strategy		Dropouts
Streznewski (1999)	Superstars	Strivers	Independents		Dropouts
Jacobsen (1999)		Balanced	Exaggerated		Collapsed
Nauta & Corten (2002)	Social	Accepted	Confrontational	Inconspicuous	Isolation
Persson (2009)	Hero		Martyr	Nerd	
Falck, current book (2020): High-IQ Relational Styles	**Thriving** (Actualising of potential)		**Provoking** (Either presumptuous of or oblivious of potential)	**Inhibited** (Holding back of potential)	**Despairing** (Disavowing of potential)

Streznewski (1999) maintains that she independently arrived at categories of giftedness outcomes that she then found matched those of psychologist Elizabeth Drews (1963). Streznewski's (1999:6) descriptors for these categories are: "strivers" ("high-testing teacher pleasers", who work hard, are career minded, and deliver reliably); "superstars" (stand out from others for excelling in various ways and for being happy); and "independents" (individuals who are seldom popular, or leaders; they are irritating to others, a problem for authorities, and don't fit into workplace systems). Streznewski then curiously mentions another category that she does not name as one of the main three, but which she acknowledges as the one "we don't like to think about" (Streznewski 1999:9). She describes this category as comprising gifted individuals who "drop out", "the ultimate waste of the best and the brightest" (Streznewski 1999:9).

Jacobsen (1999) categorises the outcomes of giftedness as depending on the person's attitude to life, what she describes as the "social strategy" that they adopt, and whether they develop skills. Her three categories are "exaggerated" (gifted abilities overwhelming the person and others, being "out of control" (Jacobsen 1999:253), and causing difficulty and negative reactions); "collapsed" (abilities being suppressed, not engaged with, causing detachment, depression, substance abuse), or "balanced" (abilities are not suppressed but are regulated, meaning that they do not overwhelm the person and are able to be well-channelled).

Nauta & Corten's (2002) categories include mention of whether the person is aware of his or her giftedness or not. Their categories are: "Inconspicuous" (low profile, restricted personal development, not aware of giftedness); "Accepted" (has established connection with others at own level, no major adaptation problems); "Social" (has actively raised social skills to a high level and can therefore solve many adaptation problems, functions well); "Confrontational" (moves from conflict to conflict and even, occupationally, from dismissal to dismissal), "Isolation" (runs the risk of losing contact with society). Something that distinguishes Nauta & Corten's contribution, is that they describe how individuals can move between the categories. So they say that an "Inconspicuous" who becomes aware of their giftedness can then develop into one of the other types, and that a "Confrontational" can progress to "Social" if social skills are developed, or can instead retreat to "Isolation".

We have already looked at Persson's (2009) work in previous chapters. So here I will just say that he explains that he is proposing a "taxonomy of gifted social functions". He theorises that "the nerd" performs the social function of societal maintenance; that "the hero" provides societal entertainment; and that "the martyr" is the one who instigates societal change.

Each of the above systems of categorisation classifies outcomes in accordance with the nature of the high-IQ/gifted individual's interpersonal relationships. Where a person is described as doing very well in terms of realising their abilities, they are also described as having interpersonal competence, for example Streznewski's "Superstars", of whom she says their concern for social relationships makes them popular with "everyone in their lives" (1999:6). At the other extreme, those who are categorised as least developing their abilities, are described in terms of interpersonal failure, such as Nauta & Corten's category of "Isolation" (2002).

Of the authors tabulated above, only Nauta & Corten (2002) use five categories, with the others using three or four. It can be seen from Table 8.1 that my framework's four quadrants map quite well onto these other authors' categories. However, those authors are fairly unknown outside of the giftedness literature. The next section relates my High-IQ Relational Styles framework to the work of various authors within mainstream psychological theory.

Congruences with other psychological thinking

Recognition revisited

Chapter 3 introduced, and Chapter 4 elaborated, the importance of the kind of recognition and interaction that takes place – or fails to take place – between the high-IQ person and his or her interpersonal environment. I highlighted Benjamin's (1995) assertion that recognition is as important to psychological survival as food is to physical survival (cited in Hollway 2015:94), and explained Winnicott's (1965; 1975) theory on the central developmental importance of experiencing mirroring from others in social interaction that validates one's sense of oneself and of being accepted by the other, thereby building self-esteem. Such mirroring enables the development of an individual's True Self (Winnicott 1975). We have such sensitivity to these early relational cues because, as has been explained, we come into the world genetically programmed to seek favourable responses from others, starting with our caregivers (Trevarthen 1979; 2001; Stern 1985), as our extreme helplessness at birth makes us entirely dependent for our survival on being protected and nurtured by another. Although as we grow and mature we develop far away from the state of literal helplessness in which our lives began, that primitive instinct of wanting to belong, together with a visceral fear of rejection or abandonment, does not disappear.

Living from one's True Self entails feeling free to express oneself authentically, and is associated with being able to be playful, creative, and to feel confident of being able to be accepted and loved (Winnicott 1971). This corresponds with the top-right "Thriving" quadrant of my High-IQ Relational Styles framework. In Winnicott's theory, a person who has not had the benefit of "good enough" mirroring/mothering (Winnicott 1952; 1975; 1988) will seek to change themselves to try to get a more favourable response from the other, and this can shut down their authentic self-expression more and more to the extent that they lose touch with their own true feelings and develop instead a "False Self" (Winnicott 1960). Living from a False Self entails trying to make oneself into someone that the other might be more likely to approve of, and is associated with feeling unreal, fake, depressed, and experiencing life as meaningless. This relates to Coleman's (2012:378) finding that "invisibility" is the most often used coping strategy of gifted youth. This corresponds with the two dark-grey shaded "Hiding Self" quadrants of my High-IQ Relational Styles framework. Winnicott explains how a person with a high IQ can be particularly susceptible to False Self development:

> A particular danger arises out of the not-infrequent tie-up between the intellectual approach and the False Self. When a False Self becomes organized in an individual who has a high intellectual potential there is a very strong tendency for the mind to become the location of the False Self, and in this case there develops a dissociation between intellectual activity and psycho-somatic existence … When there has taken place this double abnormality, (i) the False Self organized to hide the True Self, and (ii) an attempt on the part of the individual to solve the personal problem by the use of a fine intellect, a clinical picture results which is peculiar in that it very easily deceives. The world may observe academic success of a high degree, and may find it hard to believe in the very real distress of the individual concerned, who feels "phoney" the more he or she is successful. When such individuals destroy themselves in one way or another, instead of fulfilling promise, this invariably produces a sense of shock in those who have developed high hopes of the individual.
>
> *(Winnicott 1960:144)*

The tendency of gifted individuals to take flight into the intellect from challenging interpersonal demands, such as using abstraction as a regressive defence (Rosen 1958), is also documented in a study on Malaysian gifted students' coping mechanism of avoiding social difficulties by getting absorbed in academic work (Ishak & Bakar 2010).

All major theories of human development have a version of recognising the deleterious effects for well-being and mental health of living a life where one's True Self is not expressed. In Carl Rogers's Person-Centred approach, this state is termed "incongruence", and the True Self is termed the "organismic self" (Rogers 1959; 1961). With Psychoanalysis, Freud termed the attempt to get rid of the thoughts, wishes, and feelings that would draw an unfavourable response, and its resultant distortions to psychic and interpersonal life, "repression" (Freud 1915). In Eric Berne's Transactional Analysis (1961) the wish for a favourable response is termed the pursuit of "strokes". Alice Miller's (1997) book *The Drama of the Gifted Child*, is all about the expression of the True Self as being the source of self-esteem, vitality, and meaningful existence. In Attachment Theory it is secure persons who are confident of being able to express themselves authentically and gain acceptance (Bowlby 1988). Secure attachment corresponds with the top-right "Thriving" quadrant of my High-IQ Relational Styles framework. The insecurely attached person withdraws (avoidant) or exaggerates (anxious) their self-expression in an attempt to gain the most favourable response from the other. Avoidant attachment corresponds with the "Hiding Self" quadrants of my High-IQ Relational Styles framework, and anxious attachment corresponds with the bottom-right "Provoking" quadrant. What is evident in all of these major theories, is the central significance of interpersonal relationship experiences, that it is through these that one's self-image and patterns of general regular relationship behaviour get established and perpetuated (termed "internal working model" in Attachment Theory, "internal world" in Object Relations, "life position" in Transactional Analysis, and "core beliefs" in Cognitive-Behavioural Therapy).

Further considerations regarding Attachment Theory and Object Relations

The above quotation by Winnicott shows that a high-IQ person is susceptible to a "particular danger" of developing False Self functioning. My research (Falck 2013) suggested a susceptibility in high-IQ individuals to developing insecure, predominantly avoidant, attachment. Something we know about attachment is that the child's own temperament has an impact on how the caregiver relates to the child. For example, an infant who sleeps well at night and feeds unproblematically might be easier for a caregiver to relate happily and generously to than an infant who frequently fusses and appears not to be readily satisfied by the caregiver's attentions. Children with extreme intelligence, with their "hyper brain/hyper body" (Karpinski et al. 2018), can be very sensitive, intense, highly active, and strong-willed, which are traits that could make them more difficult to handle or satisfy. How the parent reacts to this will affect the child's developing character. For example, a more highly strung child who is harder to satisfy can make the mother feel inadequate, and being made to feel negatively about herself by her baby can make her feel negatively about the baby. This can in turn be experienced by the baby as the mother being less enthusiastic, confident, or satisfied with him or her. The challenges of parenting a high-IQ child might in this manner make the child more susceptible to developing insecure attachment.

Baker & Baker (1987:3) explain that children can fail to develop the "internal structures" that "regulate self-esteem" if the parent–child interaction is significantly problematic. The first reason they give for why this can occur, is that the child has "exquisite needs due to such factors as genetic predispositions, physical handicaps, or learning disabilities" – or, I would add, extreme intelligence. The second reason they give is there being "an unfortunate mismatch between the temperaments of the parent and the child" (Baker & Baker 1987:3). It is clear that the temperamental characteristics often associated with high intelligence could create a mismatch of this kind with a dissimilar parent. (The third reason they give involves the parent's own limitations such as psychopathology and/or externally imposed circumstances such as death, job loss, or illness.)

Similarly, Howe (2011) documents that there are higher proportions of insecure attachment in disabled children. Where he identifies how the difficulties that caregivers can experience in caring for a disabled child can impact on that child's developing attachment style, the factors described (such as the caregiver not understanding or being able to relate to the child's needs and therefore becoming stressed and less available to the child) could equally be true of caring for a very high-IQ child. Webb et al. (2016:95) write that many parents are "frightened, worried, confused, or even intimidated" by their "bright, strong-willed offspring". As attachment security is directly related to exploratory behaviour, high-IQ youngsters who are secure have the confidence and freedom to explore the world around them as well as their own intellects, which is conducive of actualising their potential and thriving.

Even if a high-IQ child has benefited from capable and attuned parenting, once the child reaches adolescence the primary attachment to the parents shifts and becomes centred on peer relationships. West et al. (2013) found that children who had secure attachment at 24 and 36 months had better school performance and higher IQs in middle childhood (grades 3 and 4, i.e. around age 9). Such results would lead one to expect a sample of gifted adults to show a higher proportion of secure attachment than is found in general populations. The fact that this was not the case with the gifted adults in my study (Falck 2013), with their low proportion of secure attachment and high proportion of avoidant attachment, could suggest that it is these later peer experiences that are damaging. If the gifted adolescent is unable to make the shift to secure attachments with peers because of an inability to find suitable peers, having instead an experience of not fitting in, this will be a knock to confidence and is a risk factor for developing an insecure attachment style. Research has shown that preadolescent best friend dyads are robustly correlated on measures of general intelligence (Boutwell et al. 2017). Kohut (1971) sees the failure of adequate mirroring and twinship experiences as leaving a person with a shaky sense of self, or poor self-esteem. The absence of experiencing alikeness, or twinship, with others is what so many gifted individuals are referring to when they describe their feeling of being "an outsider", not belonging, which several of my interviewees spontaneously described feeling. Silverman (2013:20) confirms how feelings of alienation "seeded" in the early years "can haunt the gifted throughout their lifespan". Mollon (2001) writes that developmental failures of this kind manifest behaviourally as a general sensitivity to disturbances of physical and psychological equilibrium and a tendency to react to these with withdrawal or rage. Withdrawal relates to the "Hiding Self" quadrants of my High-IQ Relational Styles framework, and rage relates to the "Provoking" quadrant with its underlying issue of indignation.

Summary

This chapter has presented my four-quadrant "High-IQ Relational Styles" framework, which draws together conceptually the central styles of social interaction I have discerned in my research interviews with very high-IQ individuals plus my professional practice and textual analysis of literature and research on giftedness and high IQ. The framework distils two main dimensions of interpersonal relating: expressiveness of self, and acceptance by others. For each quadrant there is a dominant interpersonal style, a dominant way of handling the high ability or potential associated with extreme intelligence, and a dominant underlying issue that fuels interactions but is often outside of conscious awareness. Two quadrants depict lower levels of expressiveness of self ("Hiding Self"), and the other two depict higher levels of expressiveness ("Reaching Out"). It has been explained how reaching out to others can be undertaken in a way that is positive or negative. Each quadrant has been explained, giving relevant examples. It has then been shown how this framework is congruent with other authors' categories of giftedness life-strategies/trajectories and with many major psychological theories.

References

Baker, H. S. & Baker, M. N. (1987). Heinz Kohut's self psychology: an overview. *American Journal of Psychiatry*, 144, pp. 1–9.

Benjamin, J. (1995). *Like Subjects, Love Objects*. New Haven, CT: Yale University Press.

Berne, E. (1961). *Transactional Analysis in Psychotherapy: A Systematic Individual and Social Psychiatry*. New York: Grove Press.

Boutwell, B. B., Meldrum, R. C. & Petkovsek, M. A. (2017). General intelligence in friendship selection: a study of preadolescent best friend dyads. *Intelligence*, 64, pp. 20–35.

Bowlby, J. (1988). *A Secure Base*. London: Routledge.

Coleman, L. J. (2012). Lived experience, mixed messages, and stigma. In: T. L. Cross & J. R. Cross (Eds.). *Handbook for Couselors Serving Students with Gifts and Talents: Development, Relationships, School Issues, and Counselling Needs/Interventions*. Waco, TX: Prufrock Press. pp. 371–392.

Corten, F., Nauta, N. & Ronner, S. (2006). *Highly intelligent and gifted employees – Key to innovation?* (English translation). Academic paper delivered in Amsterdam, 11 October 2006 at International HRD-conference. [online] Available at: www.triplenine.org/articles/Nauta-200610.pdf. [Accessed 12 June 2012].

Cross, T. L., Coleman, L. J. & Steward, R. A. (1993). The social cognition of gifted adolescents: an exploration of the stigma of giftedness paradigm. *Roeper Review*, 16(1), pp. 37–40.

Drews, E. (1963). The four faces of able adolescents. *Saturday Review of Literature*, 46, pp. 68–71.

Erikson, E. H. (1950). *Childhood and Society*. New York: W. W. Norton & Company.

Falck, S. (2013). *Attachment Styles and Experience of Workplace Interpersonal Relating in Intellectually Gifted Adults*. Unpublished Practice Evaluation Project (PEP) submitted in partial fulfilment of the requirements for the Doctorate in Psychotherapy by Professional Studies at Metanoia Institute/Middlesex University.

Favier-Townsend, A. (2014). *Perceived Causes and Long Term Effects of Delayed Academic Achievement in High IQ Adults*. Unpublished PhD thesis, University of Hertfordshire, UK.

Fiedler, E. (2012). You don't outgrow it! Giftedness across the lifespan. *Advanced Development Journal*, 13, pp. 23–41.

Fiedler, E. (2015). *Uniqueness and Belonging across the Lifespan*. Tucson, AZ: Great Potential Press.

Freeman, J. (2010). *Gifted Lives: What Happens When Gifted Children Grow Up*. London: Routledge.

Freud, S. (1915). Repression. In: *The Essentials of Psycho-Analysis*. Selected by A. Freud. Translated from the German by J. Strachey. Reprint 1991. London: Penguin Books. pp. 517–534.

Grobman, J. (2006). Underachievement in exceptionally gifted adolescents and young adults: a psychiatrist's view. *The Journal of Gifted Secondary Education*, 17, pp. 199–209.

Grobman, J. (2009). A psychodynamic psychotherapy approach to the emotional problems of exceptionally and profoundly gifted adolescents and adults: a psychiatrist's experience. *Journal for the Education of the Gifted*, 33(1), pp. 106–125.

Hollway, W. (2015). *Knowing Mothers: Researching Maternal Identity Change. Studies in the Psychosocial*. London: Palgrave Macmillan.

Howe, D. (2011). *Attachment across the Lifecourse*. New York: Palgrave Macmillan.

Ishak, N. M. & Bakar, A. Y. A. (2010). Psychological issues and the need for counselling services among Malaysian gifted students. *Procedia – Social and Behavioural Sciences*, 5, pp. 665–673.

Jacobsen, M.-E. (1999). *The Gifted Adult*. New York: Ballantine Books.

Karpinski, R. I., Kinase Kolb, A. M., Tetreault, N. A. & Borowski, T. B. (2018). High intelligence: a risk factor for psychological and physiological overexcitabilities. *Intelligence*, 66, pp. 8–23.

Kohut, H. (1971). *The Analysis of the Self*. Reprint 2009. Chicago, IL: University of Chicago Press.

Lereya, S. T., Copeland, W. E., Costello, E. J. & Wolke, D. (2015). Adult mental health consequences of peer bullying and maltreatment in childhood: two cohorts in two countries. *The Lancet*, 2(6), pp. 524–531.

Miller, A. (1997). *The Drama of the Gifted Child – The Search for the True Self*. New York: Basic Books.

Mollon, P. (2001). *Releasing the Self – The Healing Legacy of Heiz Kohut*. London: Whurr Publishers.

Nauta, N. & Corten, F. (2002). Gifted adults in work (English translation). *Tijdschrift voor Bedrijfs- en Verzekeringsgeneeeskunde* (Journal for Occupational and Insurance Physicians), 10(11), pp. 332–335. [online] Available at: www.researchgate.net/publication/319068968_Gifted_adults_in_work [Accessed 24 July 2019].

Persson, R. S. (2009). The unwanted gifted and talented: a sociobiological perspective of the societal functions of giftedness. In: L. V. Shavinina (Ed.). *International Handbook on Giftedness*. Quebec: Springer. pp. 913–924.

Peterson, J. S. & Ray, K. E. (2006a). Bullying and the gifted: victims, perpetrators, prevalence, and effects. *Gifted Child Quarterly*, 50, pp. 148–168.

Peterson, J. S. & Ray, K. E. (2006b). Bullying among the gifted: the subjective experience. *Gifted Child Quarterly*, 50, pp. 252–269.

Rogers, C. (1959). A theory of therapy, personality and interpersonal relationships as developed in the client-centered framework. In: S. Koch (Ed.). *Psychology: A Study of a Science. Vol. 3: Formulations of the Person and the Social Context*. New York: McGraw-Hill, pp. 184–256.

Rogers, C. (1961). *On Becoming a Person: A Therapist's View of Psychotherapy*. London: Constable.

Rosen, H. R. (1958). Abstract thinking and object relations: with specific reference to the use of abstraction as a regressive defence in highly gifted individuals. *Journal of the American Psychoanalytic Association*, 6(4), pp. 653–671.

Silverman, L. K. (2013). *Giftedness 101*. New York: Springer.

Stern, D. N. (1985). *The Interpersonal World of the Infant: A View from Psychoanalysis and Developmental Psychology*. New York: Basic Books.

Streznewski, M. K. (1999). *Gifted Grown Ups: The Mixed Blessings of Extraordinary Potential*. New York: John Wiley & Sons.

Towers, G. M. (1987). The outsiders. *Gift of Fire*, 22. [online] Available at: www.cpsimoes.net/artigos/outsiders.html. [Accessed 5 February 2017].

Trevarthen, C. (1979). Communication and co-operation in early infancy: a description of primary intersubjectivity. In: M. M. Bullowa (Ed.). *Before Speech: The Beginning of Interpersonal Communication*. New York: Cambridge University Press, pp. 321–347.

Trevarthen, C. (2001). Intrinsic motives for companionship in understanding: their origin, development, and significance for infant mental health. *Infant Mental Health Journal*, 22, pp. 95–131.

Webb, J. T., Amend, E. R., Beljan, P., Webb, N. E., Kuzujanakis, M., Olenchak, F. R. & Goerss, J. (2016). *Misdiagnosis and Dual Diagnoses of Gifted Children and Adults*. (2nd ed.). Tucson, AZ: Great Potential Press.

West, K. K., Mathews, B. I. & Kerns, K. A. (2013). Mother-child attachment and cognitive performance in middle childhood: an examination of mediating mechanisms. *Early Childhood Research Quarterly*, 28, pp. 259–270.

Winnicott, D. W. (1952). Letter to Roger Money-Kyrle, 27th November. In: D. W. Winnicott & F. R. Rodman (Eds.). 1987. *The Spontaneous Gesture: Selected Letters of D.W. Winnicott*. London: Karnac. pp. 38–43.

Winnicott, D. W. (1960). Ego distortion in terms of true and false self. In D. W. Winnicott (Ed.). *The Maturational Processes and the Facilitating Environment*. Reprint 1990. London: Karnac. pp. 140–152.

Winnicott, D. W. (1965). *The Maturational Processes and the Facilitating Environment*. Reprint 2005. London: Karnac.

Winnicott, D. W. (1971). *Playing and Reality*. New York: Routledge Classics.

Winnicott, D. W. (1975). *Collected Papers: Through Paediatrics to Psycho-Analysis*. London: Tavistock Publications.

Winnicott, D. W. (1988). *Babies and Their Mothers*. London: Free Association Books.

Yermish, A. (2010). *Cheetahs on the Couch: Issues Affecting the Therapeutic Working Alliance with Clients Who Are Cognitively Gifted*. Unpublished PhD thesis, Massachusetts School of Professional Psychology.

9
HELPING HIGH ABILITY THRIVE
Channelling abilities whilst managing threat

> **Reflective Prompt 9:** If you wanted to do well in a competitive environment, would your assumption be that it would be best for you to work independently or best to collaborate with others? Can you identify some factors that have influenced you in making that assumption? If you had to advise a highly able person on how best to fulfil their potential whilst ensuring their well-being, what three top tips would you emphasise to them? Why?

Part II of the book explored difficulties and dangers associated with very high IQ, and now this final chapter of Part III focuses on how we might best be able to facilitate its thriving: how can we nurture healthy psychosocial development around extreme intelligence? "Threat" in the chapter's title refers to all the risks to well-being that extreme intelligence can make a person vulnerable to. Interpersonally, it is the threat that high-IQ individuals can experience of being rejected on the basis of how they conduct and express themselves, which can make them give up on trying to express themselves, and it also relates to the threat they can pose to others. For example, functioning that is impressively fast and complex can cause others to feel "left behind", inadequate in their own ability, and insecure that the high-IQ person might in some way that matters to them, supersede them. Others can resultingly withdraw from an extremely intelligent person or become hostile or obstructive because of feeling disconcerted and/or threatened by him or her.

This chapter distils some basic guiding principles regarding how to manage some of these threats or risks – in parenting and schooling, in the workplace, and in personal performance – so that high ability can be engaged with rather than wasted. The chapter also presents – with reference to the High-IQ Relational Styles framework – the change process that is involved in moving towards the "Thriving" quadrant, with mention of relevant resources. It ends by reflecting on what is meant by "success".

Parenting and schooling

Issues to do with parenting and schooling have been referred to throughout the book, with more specific detail around the challenges of parenting an extremely intelligent child contained in the latter part of Chapter 6 (from the "Misdiagnosis" section onwards) and in the final section of Chapter 8. The main principles that these sections indicate are the importance of a) identifying what is being dealt with; b) accessing relevant resources that can provide information about and appropriate support with the issues involved; and c) developing effective strategies for dealing with the issues. Each of these will be discussed below. None of this is an exact science, so flexibility, imagination, and an acceptance of diversity are needed in order to respond optimally to different individuals within their different individual circumstances, which will include all the environmental variables of country, culture, family, and what educational and occupational opportunities are available. Trial and error are likely to be necessary to forge a path that works best for any particular child. Maintaining a strengths-based perspective is empowering, but should not be used to deny the reality of difficulties and struggles that are involved.

Identification

Identifying extreme intelligence in a child involves noticing signs of high sensitivity and intensity emotionally, physically, and intellectually: this includes – as a rudimentary summary – high curiosity, concentration, and wilfulness; and performance in motor skill, learning, and creativity that is of a maturity beyond what is expected for his or her age. It is to be remembered, however, that children who have twice/dual/multiple exceptionality might not manifest all of these traits: there might be high intelligence coupled with, for example, dysgraphia, which is one kind of exception (in that case, to motor skill proficiency), and therefore an alertness to the complexity of different possible presentations and variations is necessary. The development of such a child might proceed fairly seamlessly if these traits are engaged with well by parents and educational environments that are responsive and peers who are compatible. This is aided by early detection of high ability, which Silverman (2013) stresses as essential for optimal development. Signs that extreme intelligence might be present but not adequately engaged with can arise in boredom, frustration, disruptive behaviour, and low attainment. In a more timid or compliant child such signs can be subtle. However, when such signs are not attended to they can escalate into anxiety, depression, and worse. If these sorts of difficulties manifest in any child then extreme intelligence as one of the possible causes should be held in mind.

Formal identification of extreme intelligence such as IQ testing might never be required if the associated traits are being well responded to and engaged with as described above. Even if difficulties do arise, such testing is unnecessary if the nature of the difficulties can be ascertained and adequately resolved. However, where difficulties persist, formal IQ testing can be a helpful diagnostic tool towards building understanding of what issues are involved. For example, identifying that there are significant discrepancies between scores in verbal and non-verbal IQ can be useful for understanding what a child might be struggling with and therefore how best to assist him or her. Additional testing might be necessary to assess for other potential conditions such as dyslexia if dual or multiple exceptionality is suspected.

Another – more systemic – aspect of assessment, is identifying what the parents of such a child might be struggling with. Given the high genetic transmission of intelligence, the issues involved are likely to have affected the parent/s also, and sometimes the first time that the parents start to identify how this relates to themselves is when they are confronted with having to deal with how it relates to their child. With this can come a stirring up of complicated memories of how intelligence was, in their own childhoods, perhaps suppressed or over-emphasised. Related attitudes and assumptions can be completely unconsciously repeated towards their own children.

A further point to recognise is that insofar as high intelligence can sometimes correlate with features of autism, if the parent/s themselves are thus affected they might not be in a position to identify social interaction nuances in their child and help them understand and deal with these. If a child's academic performance at school is adequate he or she might get by without the deficits he or she is suffering from in social interaction ever being taken seriously. I have had clients who went through their whole childhoods without this being identified, but then in young adulthood – when expected to be able to manage on their own with finding friends, partners, and occupations – they started having significant difficulties with establishing or sustaining any or all of these and only then started paying specific attention to this.

Resources

As can be seen from the above section and indeed all the previous chapters, what is of enormous help in successfully nurturing extreme intelligence is finding environments that have differentiated provision that is specifically suitable for very high-IQ individuals and where they can experience themselves as belonging with similar others rather than conspicuously standing out as different. Grobman (2009) writes about how helpful it can be for gifted individuals to find ways of seeing themselves as ordinary, even though they are in some respects exceptional. For a child who is functioning intellectually at two or more standard deviations above the level that average mixed-ability schools are pitched at, the question of how best to provide for him or her educationally is pivotal. This is the single most prevalent issue in the literature and research on giftedness, filling numerous journals, conferences and books, and occupying several organisations internationally.

The main ways that extreme intelligence is dealt with in childhood education is by ignoring it in ordinary mixed-ability schools that have no differentiated provision; such schools offering occasional enrichment classes or enrichment classes having to be accessed in extracurricular programmes; grade acceleration; selective schools; or home-schooling. Entering into the pros and cons of each of these is far beyond what we have space for here, but these can be researched within whichever geographical region is applicable. However, whichever of these approaches is considered, a couple of main principles are relevant.

A first principle is to be alert to two main different thinking styles: auditory-sequential (preferring to receive information in verbal, linear form, focusing on facts and details) or visual-spatial (thinking primarily in images, seeking a holistic overview) (see Webb et al. 2016). Identifying and accepting a learner's preferences and adapting activities accordingly can transform engagement with learning. An allied principle is that highly structured education causes lower performance in high-IQ students because they lose interest and motivation: this was evidenced clearly with the SMPY participants (Hunt 2011:346). Allowing leeway for self-direction and autonomy in learning is what is most conducive of thriving.

Giftedness – like creativity – is associated with divergent thinking, which is the opposite of structured, rational, concretely focused activity. It is divergent thinking that characterises the dreaminess in Elon Musk (see Chapter 6) that confounded those around him. This is prominent also in the girl hailed as the new contemporary Mozart – Alma Deutscher – who is home-schooled and given freedom to live in her imagination, where prolific musical creations come to her as she jumps daily with her treasured skipping rope (Williams 2017). Traditional Western schooling is not conducive of such processes and prioritises logico-rational convergent thinking, rewarding (such as with higher grades) those who can operate in that way. The giving of grades emphasises outcome rather than process, and external validation rather than an internally directed passion and motivation together with a personal evaluation of learning needs, progress, and achievement. It also exacerbates rivalry. The school Elon Musk founded in 2014 to educate his own children – called Ad Astra, meaning "to the stars" – does not use grades.

Strategies: safeguarding against naivety and arrogance

The very beginning of any parenting involves establishing and then maintaining intersubjective attunement between parent and child – otherwise known as bonding. This is the medium for all the interpersonal mirroring and co-regulation of affect that has been referred to in previous chapters. Probably one of the most pernicious contemporary parenting practices is putting a demanding or distressed child in front of a screen (television, tablet, phone, etc.) in hope of thereby removing the problem. The more that such a strategy dominates the more it will actually exacerbate the problem, because being distracted by an interactive digital device rather than being provided with an interactive human caregiver ultimately breeds anxiety as the child does not learn how to identify and articulate his or her own emotional states or those of others, or learn how to manage these interpersonally, or learn how to effectively seek and find comfort from others. If a parent lacks confidence as to how to provide attuned interaction, help is available: one technology-free resource for bonding with, playing with, and providing affect-regulation with a child, is Theraplay (Booth 2010), which has an evidence base for effectiveness including where autism is involved (Hiles Howard et al. 2018).

In cases where marked ability and/or difficulty becomes apparent in a child, what needs to be avoided in any assessment process and outcome is treatment of the child that is fearful, overawed, overindulging, or pressurising. An overarching principle of maintaining balance is key, whereby the child's abilities are neither ignored and neglected nor unduly exalted. In tandem with the principle of balance, is the essential point of needing to show children that they are valued – as well as held accountable for their behaviour – completely independently of whatever they might or might not be able to achieve. Another well-documented principle to remember is not to praise intelligence as though it is a fixed entity but to encourage a growth-oriented mindset by endorsing effort (Dweck 2006).

Interpersonal responses to extreme intelligence optimally require a balance between engaging with, and providing containment for, the – at times challenging – characteristics involved of high energy, pronounced sensitivity and curiosity, and strong will. Providing containment means establishing boundaries that are clearly communicated and reliably adhered to. Such containment should not, however, hurt, humiliate, or "clip the wings" of the individual. Without such containment, gifted individuals can experience overstimulation, emotional flooding, and a sense of endless possibilities and grandiose personal power, together with feeling bad about themselves and unsafe in relation to others when people describe them as "scary" or "frighteningly smart" (Grobman 2009). Benjamin (cited in Hollway 2015) states that you need someone to come up against you, match you, not let you get away with things. Grobman found that his patients "began to realise that their larger-than-life successes did not mean that they lived outside the boundaries of human nature or were exempt from its laws" (2009:116), and that "the normal parameters of conflict resolution still applied to them".

It is fundamental, therefore, for healthy development that realistic boundaries are provided that bring about an experience for the child of being gradually frustrated in his or her most selfish demands, but not beyond what the child can developmentally manage, so as not to cause trauma but to foster increasing tolerance and a growing ability to manage the self by internalising such realistic boundaries. This allows the child to gradually become more independent (Mollon 2001) and self-disciplined as well as respectful of others. In this way a child is safeguarded against developing arrogance. When gifted individuals do not experience a developmentally suitable boundary that they can respect, this can lead to them having problems with authority and even to finding themselves within the criminal justice system, as documented in Chapter 4's section "From the classroom to the courtroom". However, if boundaries are provided to high-IQ children in an authoritarian way, where their individuality and the value of the contribution they can make is not validated and their need for autonomy is not respected, this can be very damaging for them – more so than for average-IQ youngsters – and may affect their mental health (Yazdani & Daryei 2016).

Talking openly with children in an age-appropriate way about the issues involved – thereby imparting psychoeducation and assisting them to construct an effective vocabulary around intrapersonal feelings and experiences and interpersonal behaviours and skills – safeguards against naivety. Fundamental to carrying this out is effective communication. Many resources can be drawn on to assist with this, two of which are Fonseca (2016) and Peters (2018).

In the workplace: facilitating collaboration and competition

In adulthood it is often the workplace that provides the arena within which the channelling of abilities and the fulfilling (or not) of potential is grappled with. As mentioned in Chapter 6, there is literature suggesting that the very fact of being extremely intelligent can impede a person's career progress. Perrone et al. (2004:128) found that for academically talented individuals, the second highest perceived barrier to career success (after commitment to non-work roles) was "organizational politics or interpersonal relationships in the work environment". Not being able to work effectively with others can certainly be a hindrance because, just as combinatorial thought (see Chapter 6; Simonton 2009) is the most productive kind, which integrates different mental processes within one individual's mind, so combinatorial collaborations between two or more individuals can enormously extend the fecundity and reach of purely solitary endeavour. Workplace interpersonal issues and difficulties associated with gifted adults are cited by many authors (Jacobsen 1999; Streznewski 1999; De Raat 2002; Nauta & Corten 2002; Corten et al. 2006; Persson 2009; Nauta & Ronner 2013). However, general workplace-related literature focuses on the pragmatics of how to cope with difficult behaviour (e.g. Weeks 2008; Kusy & Holloway 2009), or how to increase emotional intelligence (e.g. Goleman 1998; Tan 2012), rather than on identifying or understanding underlying causes of difficulty such as the individual differences associated with the neuroatypicality of very high IQ.

A multinational company that specifically thinks about the underlying causes of workplace friction and that has created a business model based on emphasising neuroatypicality, is Auticon, who provide IT consulting services but only employ as consultants individuals who are on the autistic spectrum. I attended a fascinating evening hosted by Mensa which brought together Auticon, their investor Virgin, and CRAE (the UCL Institute of Education's Centre for Research in Autism and Education). I saw in the presentations how similar the interpersonal difficulties are that high-IQ/gifted adults, and autistic adults, encounter in neurotypical-dominant workplaces. Such difficulties include struggling with small talk and office politics, offending others with their bluntness, and getting frustrated at others' lack of attention to detail. Auticon places their consultants in the work teams of major corporations after using specially trained job coaches to brief the team and prepare the work environment to be suitable for the autistic consultant's needs. The agreement is that when difficulties arise, the employer does not raise it with the consultant, but contacts the job coach, who hears what has happened and "decodes" the differences that caused a problem, interpreting the autistic person's functioning to the employer and assisting the employer to better assimilate into their work practices the characteristics presented by autism. The exemplary feature of Auticon is that it is entirely accepting of the way the autistic person functions and it works to help environments understand that and interact with that more constructively, rather than trying to change the autistic person's way of being. This highlights the question of what sort of intervention is best for facilitating different environments and neuroatypical individuals to harness the strengths that such diverse individuals offer, for their mutual benefit.

My very high-IQ interviewees did stress what a difference was made by the kinds of structure and culture of the workplaces they had experienced. The importance of the right organisational fit for gifted workers is also highlighted by Menel (2008). Interviewees most disliked – describing it as the worst aspect of their job or the reason for leaving a job – hierarchical systems where, as Harry described,

> If you don't have grey hair then … it's deemed that you are less knowledgeable than the person who has had more years' experience …

Interviewees most thrived in systems where autonomy, creativity, and initiative were encouraged rather than orders being expected to be followed, and where contributions were welcomed on their own merits regardless of status. The best workplace cultures were those that supported free communication without hierarchical restriction, promoting open but respectful feedback focused on the betterment of the task at hand rather than on practices driven by individuals building and protecting their own egos and power bases. Where interviewees described their workplaces as comprising environments that in these ways showed a welcoming of and employing of gifted ability, such interviewees described enjoying high levels of job satisfaction, feeling they were using their full potential, and having fewer experiences of obstruction and more experiences of positive collaboration.

Experiences of obstruction were often connected with competition: as documented in Chapters 4 and 5, high ability that poses a threat to someone else's power attracts attempts to thwart it. For example, when Avi at his own initiative developed a full report on an opportunity his company could expand into, he was criticised: "That's not what we've hired you for". This is like the myth of Arachne who boasted she could weave better than the goddess Athena. They entered into a competition, in which it started becoming apparent that Arachne was indeed better. However, Athena was more powerful. She retaliated by transforming Arachne into a relegated life form – a spider, whose stunningly woven webs would forevermore be summarily dusted away as a nuisance. Learning wisdom about how to display what you are capable of, so as to keep yourself safe in relation to the powers around you, is what interviewee Wayne described:

> In an interview, if you look too confident you come across as a threat. You have to try and portray yourself as having less knowledge than they do and not being as clever as they are, almost like being a dog that's subservient to its master, you've got to display the attitude where, I find, always make them aware they can pat you down, keep you on the leash.

Jane said that "people feel insecure that someone clever has come along because they will of course use that cleverness to get ahead", and losing out to someone else is what "anybody fears". Competition can, of course – as long as it is not annihilating in its threat – be a powerfully productive adversarial force that stimulates higher motivation, innovation and achievement.

Most interviewees had become known at work for their capability which had resulted in them taking up helping roles of one kind or another. Some described helping others as bringing them enjoyment, self-esteem, and providing enhancement of their own learning. Jane expressed the idea that:

> ... if you have a gift, you have an intelligence, or you're born with a high social status, you have a moral obligation to use it for the benefit of others.

However, frustration could be felt when others sought their help rather than finding out for themselves. Or, they could try to help but become impatient, and some preferred not to be in the helper role, or – as Hans specified – not with people below a certain minimum level of skill. And Erik mentioned that one could be more productive in advancing one's own work when not having to spend time helping others.

My interviewees talked about how much their productivity increased when working with colleagues who had similar abilities to their own. They described such colleagues as being ones who "are quick to understand things" and "can make really relevant input themselves" (Erik); with whom "you can really make things spark and create a chemistry" (Helene); who are "stimulating and inspiring" and with whom it is possible to "challenge each other in all sorts of ways" (Mei). Such collaboration was described as absolutely exhilarating:

> Really bouncing off ideas and it was this ... you know, here's an idea. I would criticise and say, "Yeah, that's great, but what about this?" And then you know ... we eventually got the solution and it was fantastic. And I don't think we could have done it alone.
>
> *(Hans)*

> What do I love most about it? The moment when it's all come together and you're on the stage and you've got an orchestra and colleagues and an audience. And you get so involved in what you're doing and it's almost like you cease to be you and you're getting the feedback from the audience. And you're giving that energy out to them and it just ... it's a symbiosis. It's wonderful ... It's ... It's an awful cliché, but it's like flying. You stop being grounded, just for a bit. Try feeling grounded when you've got a 65-piece orchestra underneath you!
>
> *(Helene)*

Revisiting High-IQ Relational Styles: change towards "Thriving"

Chapter 3 ended by outlining three kinds of change that could be attempted if a very high-IQ person was experiencing difficulty in achieving their goals: first, trying to change the nature of the person; second, changing the nature of the environment; or third, making change in the interface between the person and the environment, i.e. changing the person's way of interacting with their environment. How this relates to the High-IQ Relational Styles framework is described below and depicted in Figure 9.1. As explained at the end of Chapter 8, in the High-IQ Relational Styles framework it is the "Thriving" quadrant that represents optimal functioning, and therefore what would be viewed as beneficial change would be change that moves towards the way of functioning that is represented in that "Thriving" quadrant.

It can be said that the first kind of change – trying to change the nature of the person – incorporates the High-IQ Relational Styles framework's two left-hand-side "Hiding Self" quadrants, because holding back on one's potential ("Inhibited") or disavowing one's potential ("Despairing") both involve trying to change one's nature. Such a change involves a decreasing of expressiveness of self, and creating a False Self, as opposed to fully developing and expressing

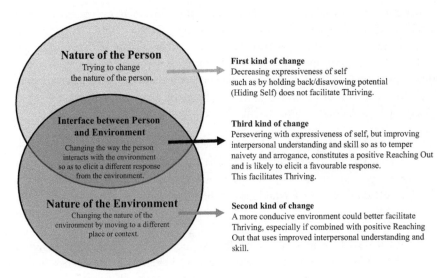

FIGURE 9.1 Change towards "Thriving"

one's True Self. This constitutes the opposite of the freedom and actualisation that characterises the "Thriving" quadrant. Trying to change the nature of the person is therefore not an advocated form of change, and for that reason will not be discussed below.

The second kind of change – changing one's environment by moving to a different place or context – can be beneficial if this effects a better person-environment fit. However, even if an environment is more conducive, the person's way of interacting with the environment will still always have an impact on outcomes.

The third kind of change – changing one's way of interacting with the environment – could involve trying to achieve one's goals by indignantly demanding from others ("Provoking") in a manner that is naive or arrogant. That would constitute a "Reaching Out" to others that is negative as it would be more likely to alienate others and not help with achieving one's goals. Alternatively, change could be undertaken that involves persevering with an expressiveness of self (rather than "Hiding Self"), but by interacting with the environment in a way that tempers both naivety and arrogance so as not to be "Provoking". This would involve a "Reaching Out" that is positive as it would be likely to elicit a favourable response from others and improve well-being, interpersonal relating, and an actualising of potential. In other words, this would be a change that would aid an entering into of the "Thriving" quadrant. And even if a change of environment is undertaken, a practice of positive "Reaching Out" to others will augment one's prospects of "Thriving" within the new environment.

The first part of the change process is a perceiving of something as being significantly unsatisfactory, or a glimpsing of a significantly desirable potential, which provides motivation for a change. This is followed by a decision at some level to make a change, then an actual implementing of the decision: I say a decision "at some level" because this whole process, or any component of it, can vary as to how accessible it is to conscious awareness.

Changing the nature of the environment

As shown in Chapter 3, because of the differences in different kinds of environment, it might mean that moving to a different place or context enables improved well-being, interpersonal relating, and actualising of potential. A few interviewees described very different experiences in different environments, like Gill (change from comprehensive to grammar school), Erik (change of workplace), and Hans (change of culture in different school in a different country). Sometimes such a move of location would be instigated by glimpsing a significantly desirable potential elsewhere, as happened with Ana:

> [Describing a trip to London] After about five days I fell in love with myself and I was quite surprised, and I tried to analyse what was the reason and I figured out that the behaviour of people here, the cultural context means that … no one ever said, "Oh that's weird, we don't do that", or, "How can you?". No one criticised, no one made me feel awkward or wrong, and by just treating me as if everything I do or think or say is okay it did something to me … and I thought, "If people behave like that and I need a good energy to understand who I am, I need to move there".

Experiencing something different created for her the fantasy of London as a better place, which she then tried to make real by moving to London. Other interviewees also talked about a fantasy of a better place, whether or not it was something they had managed to realise. For example, Wayne harboured the fantasy that if he'd grown up in communist Russia "I would have been singled out and the government would have made something of me". Helene described how she felt as an adolescent:

> I wanted to go to America … I wanted more than anything to get out of New Zealand …Too small. Too far away from everywhere. Too dismissive of anything intellectual or cultural.

Webb et al. (2016) also write about how a gifted adult might travel to locate peers more similar to themselves and access more suitable educational or occupational opportunities. However, as pointed out in Chapter 3, changing environments might not always be possible. Even where it is possible, it can be a costly procedure logistically, financially, and emotionally, with uncertain success: if you keep doing exactly what you always have done you might find that it works better in a changed environment, but it might be that the same problems will recur in the new environment.

Change in the interface between self and environment

Making constructive changes to the way one interacts with the environment – in other words, reaching out to others in a way that is positive, that tempers naivety and arrogance and is not provoking – essentially means improving interpersonal understanding and skill. The majority of my interviewees described changes they had exerted specific effort to effect as a result of their learning about what had caused interpersonal difficulty and their wish to make their interpersonal relating better. Changes were implemented for personal reasons (such as wanting friends and a partner) or professional reasons (such as seeking more effective work collaborations). Avi emphasised that in his experience social skills were much more important for work success than anything else such as qualifications. Sean spoke of regretting his lack of focus on social skills as he realised, now that he had his own business, how helpful it would be if he had in previous years been more mindful of developing social networks that he could now draw upon.

Don described how the change process occurred for him, instigated by what he was experiencing as a significantly unsatisfactory situation of having had "very few friends", and not managing to relate to girls. He noticed "people developing social skills naturally. For me they never came naturally". He described reading the article "The Outsiders" (Towers 1987):

> It's about this guy who is the most intelligent person ever, IQ of 220, and then at three years old he taught himself Greek, and then at 16 he decided to be celibate, he never married, he never had children ... So I could actually understand him, it's like a breakdown. The world is cruel and big and if you try to do this attitude, "I'm right, the world is wrong", it's the end.
> ... I had this feeling that I wanted to be normal, and people will say I'm weird and it would really hurt me ... I have always wanted to be a normal person in the sense that having a normal job, having a girl. Now I'm immensely proud of being brave and saying, "I was an arsehole, I want to change". It's something that takes a long time and it's very difficult, but now I'm very normal, I don't have any health problems, I have many friends, I'm doing well at the office.

Rather than withdrawing and giving up in the way that William James Sidis did, who is the person referred to in the article, the change that Don made entailed reaching out to others by specifically working to improve his interpersonal skill. The article explains Sidis as having withdrawn because of the painfulness – or trauma – of his childhood, and he also dropped out from developing his potential, which fits my "Despairing" quadrant. However, a person might be celibate, unmarried, or childless not because of trauma but because of personal preference, and these are respect-worthy choices. If, however, a person is not making such choices out of preference, but is struggling to secure the kind of relationships they are longing for – as was the case with interviewee Don – then that is where finding healing of trauma and developing interpersonal skill can assist.

One such skill that several interviewees described – in contrast with a more pervasive "Hiding Self" manner of shutting down one's natural way of being – involved a consciously employed and temporary situational holding back of themselves, such as knowing an answer but not giving it. Mei likened her experience to the film *Groundhog Day*, where "you already see the ending", "you know what to expect", but you "sit back and let the event unfold itself" so as to encourage others to contribute rather than rushing ahead with the conclusion yourself. Deliberately choosing to hold back on certain things at certain times means also being able to lift the control and be fully expressive of self when the context is appropriate. Another skill that some interviewees mentioned was the use of humour to dissipate or smooth over interpersonal difficulties:

> … one thing I try … is to be humorous, and I think I'm gifted to that extent that I can crack jokes and find humour in different situations, like making impressions of people and how they might say in so and so situation, and my work colleagues find that very, very funny, which is great and once you crack up somebody it breaks the ice …
>
> *(Avi)*

What the changes made in interpersonal relating most frequently involved were the following:

1. Gaining a better understanding of individual differences: not everybody has the same capacities you have.
2. Accordingly adapting the way you operate so as to a) temper what does come naturally (which often involves having to slow yourself down) or b) augment what does not come naturally (appreciating the value in all others, and developing awareness of their perspectives and how they might be experiencing you).
3. Making specific attempts to be more inclusive of others.
4. Having to keep on investing in all of the above: interviewees spoke of the effort that was needed to bring about improvement in interpersonal skill, and of how continuing effort was needed in order to sustain improvements.

The essence of these insights is contained in Fonagy et al.'s (2004) term "mentalisation", introduced in Chapter 6. Mentalisation refers to the recognition that we all have minds, and minds that are different from each other's; that what we have in mind influences our behaviour; and that we are constantly being affected by – and are interpreting – each other's behaviour. It has been evidenced (Fonagy et al. 2004) that interpersonal relating improves with increasing skill at mentalisation, meaning a deliberate taking into account of and active practising of mentalisation. Something else to remember is what has been explicated in Chapter 7 about unconscious processes, and how becoming aware of and challenging transference, valency, and repetition compulsion is important for generating change.

Resources that interviewees mentioned as having made a difference for them, assisting in their change process, included role models, books, and feedback from others (Don); coaching at work (Don, Mei); convening a group where social skills could be taught and learning could take place from each other within the group (Avi); insight from a friend (Erik); therapy (Ana, John); seeking and finding a like-minded friendship group (Helene, Jane, Max); and a "rescuing" romantic relationship (Tracy). Bonnie had a more dramatic input into her change process, through an institutional stay: she spent four years in prison where she also had therapy and participated in groups. As she gave birth to her first child whilst in prison, she was incarcerated within a special mother-and-baby unit. In that very contained environment she experienced the expert psychotherapeutic support she received with bonding with and parenting her developing baby – in tandem with being supported to develop herself – as transformative.

Something that all of these experiences of helpful assistance have in common is that they involved relational learning and healing that acted upon what in essence had involved relational difficulty or even trauma: the trauma or difficulty that has come about in the realm of relationships is best healed through relationship. In other words, interpersonal difficulty (rupture) improves through attentive interpersonal engagement (repair) (see Schore 2012). For my interviewees, the interpersonal repair that took place occurred within either personal or professional relationships, in a one-to-one setting (with friends, colleagues, romantic partners, therapists, coaches), and/or group settings (remedial and therapy groups, networking and skills sharing groups, friendship groups). In the case of interviewee Hugh, he described how meeting together with a group of friends to play niche board games every weekend in adolescence honed his interpersonal skill in ways that became directly applicable to his later career as a senior executive on corporate boards.

It was apparent how much the interviewees valued successful interpersonal relating. For example, Hugh said that he takes particular pride in the fact that throughout his life he has only lost one friend. When I asked John what he was most proud of or most pleased with in his life so far, he replied "Undoubtedly my relationship with my spouse".

For movement to take place towards the "Thriving" quadrant from any of the other three quadrants, the issues underlying those quadrants need to be addressed (i.e. guilt, trauma, or indignance), whether this is identified and done at a conscious level, or whether the reparative interpersonal experience attends to the issue without it ever being specifically named. So, for example, interviewee Tracy described how a partner "saved" her at a time when she had very much "closed off" ("Despairing"). This romantic relationship gradually won her trust and gave her the experience of a level of acceptance that healed previous interpersonal trauma and facilitated her to begin to flourish. Finally experiencing being fully accepted is what changed everything for her.

I have heard many high-IQ adults describe how much more able they were to be tolerant and accepting of others, quelling their indignation, once they experienced themselves as being understood and accepted. Sometimes it was just having their unusually high IQ identified, whether formally or informally, that made all the difference, making sense of the difficult disparities they had experienced between themselves and others, and suddenly enabling them to relate to that experience differently and more positively. Very often they had taken the difficulties they experienced between themselves and others as meaning that there was something wrong with themselves. For example, many have described that they started thinking they must be very stupid because other people were not understanding something that they saw as so simple that they then started thinking the only explanation must be that the other people were seeing a layer of complexity that they themselves were too stupid to be seeing. The helpfulness of this process of coming to understand what is causing the difficulties between self and others, in a way that augments one's own self-esteem, is also described by Streznewski (1999) and Jacobsen (1999). Grobman (2009) has detailed how psychotherapy enabled unconscious guilt to be identified and worked through, setting gifted individuals free to actualise their potential rather than holding themselves back, hiding themselves, or sabotaging their development.

Making the kinds of changes in interpersonal relating that are described above resulted in the interviewees becoming much more attuned to their impact on others. As Tess put it, "I'm very like *uber* sensitive about saying the right and the wrong thing to people". It was acknowledged, though, how difficult the sustaining of such changes could be. This was put candidly and amusingly by Don:

> … you always get this feeling that, "Oh I'm the best … I want to be the boss of everybody". You have to fight with it … We always still have this inner baby saying, "I'm very clever, I'm always right".

Professional consultancy resources: therapy, coaching

Relationships as a resource have been described so far as being able to be reparative, but relationships could also be experienced as inadequate, or at worst harming. Interviewee Ana spoke about a bad experience of therapy, where she felt the therapist was not able to understand her and be responsive to her needs, and how this significantly increased her distress. Tess talked about an experience of coaching at work that was ineffectual through being far too simplistic. In the UK there is currently no training to prepare therapists or coaches for working effectively with the special needs of extremely intelligent individuals. In the *Handbook of Evidence-Based Psychotherapies* (Freeman & Power 2007), in the section titled "Psychological Treatment of Disorder and Specific Client Groups", there is a chapter on "Intellectual Disabilities". In delineating their topic the authors of this chapter write:

> One always wonders whether it would be seen as transparently ridiculous if one were to write a chapter on the evidence base for treatments developed for members of MENSA *[sic]*, the society for those with superior intellect. (Do we detect one or two of you raising an eyebrow at the possibility of a new research field?) Similarly, no one is looking for a cure for giftedness.
>
> *(Lindsay & Sturney 2007:193)*

This quotation demonstrates an acceptance that such a thing as "superior intellect" or "giftedness" does exist, but shows ignorance about this field together with an assumption that it is "transparently ridiculous" to think there is any relevance in researching or developing expertise to work professionally with this individual difference as a specific client group. This attitude probably derives from another typical assumption, which is that people with "superior intellect" are fine, privileged even (as the unfortunate term "gifted" suggests), and will inevitably do well. We have seen by now that this assumption is by no means accurate. Intelligence being something that is rarely talked about means that psychotherapists do not consider it as a dimension of individual difference that could be affecting a client's life, and correspondingly it does not occur to them to initiate or facilitate discussion of this. I have seen students and supervisees grapple with issues that from the perspective of my knowledge base are related to the psychosocial implications of extreme intelligence, but which they have not been in a position to be able to identify. As with any personal issue that has pertinence to be engaged with therapeutically, the starting point in preparing practitioners to be able to competently address it professionally is for them to explore their own personal history with it and their reactions to – and assumptions and attitudes about – this topic, which is what the current book's Reflective Prompts have invited.

There is a growing literature on the need for specialist understanding and skill in therapists to equip them to work effectively with gifted clients (Peterson & Moon 2008; Grobman 2009; Yermish 2010; Silverman 2013; Peterson 2015). Just as there is speculation in gifted education about whether "it takes one to teach one", there is speculation about what kind of practitioner might work most effectively with gifted clients. It has been documented that a high-ability client is susceptible to leaving therapy prematurely if the therapist does not "get" giftedness (Grobman 2009; Yermish 2010).

A practitioner such as a coach or therapist might find it particularly challenging to be confronted with a gifted client – see, for example, the article *Help ... My Client is Brilliant! Coaching People with High IQs* (Gordon, n.d.). So many people in helping professions go into these roles with a (sometimes unconscious) assumption that they will be "better off" than those who they are setting out to help, and that this is what "qualifies" them to be in a position to be of help. It can therefore be difficult when, contrary to this expectation, practitioners encounter instead a client whose functioning is so advanced that it might exceed their own, and when – whatever the client's specific difficulties might be – the "fruits" of the client's life (in responsibilities, lifestyle, connections, opportunities, wealth, status) might be impressive and enviable. A practitioner who is not prepared for this could react by feeling intimidated, inadequate, and de-skilled. The risk is then very much present of compassion breakdown (see Chapter 4's section, "The dynamics of envy: a compassion barrier"). At worst, such a practitioner might get caught in a kind of power struggle with the client, trying to assert authority in the relationship, or might reassure him- or herself of having expertise to offer that the client is in need of by in some way almost emphasising the client's deficits rather than working to build his or her strengths. Such countertransferential responses might remain unconscious and go unexamined even in supervision unless the professionals concerned have some alertness to these issues.

Yermish (2010) points out that in conducting psychotherapy with gifted adults, it can be surprising how rapidly they can make progress. In the course of my research I noticed how much use my extremely intelligent participants were able to make of even that one research interview. One example is that Gill started independently – completely unprompted – coming to an awareness and shift in perspective during the interview, just by being facilitated to talk reflectively about her experiences. During the interview she clearly came to realise how much the trauma and caution from her early years (described in Chapter 7) were still affecting her life, and towards the end of the interview she spontaneously said, "Thinking about it like this and going through it has made me realise really that's my main problem at work, is that I probably shouldn't be quite so afraid to show what I can do I suppose". Several interviewees in their feedback on their experience of participating in the research said that they had found it "therapeutic".

Optimising personal performance

As mentioned above, whatever might be extraordinary about individuals who have extreme intelligence, they are not exempt from the laws of human nature. They still need suitable nutrition to fuel their endeavour. Their cognitive performance – like anyone's – will be aided by keeping well hydrated (Fadda et al.

2012). The importance of sleep applies to them too. Without regular exercise they will not be in good physical shape. Paul Dirak – a quantum pioneer who is regarded as one of the most significant physicists of the 20th century – was famous for taking regular long walks (Farmelo 2009). Alan Turing – in between all of his stellar achievements – was a dedicated marathon runner (Hodges 2014). Steve Jobs swore by yoga (Isaacson 2011).

Turing said that he ran to relieve stress. The well-documented deleterious effects of stress mean that having a reliable stress-relief strategy is essential for maintaining health. In addition to good nutrition, sleep, and exercise, another evidenced method of reducing stress is practising meditation (Chiesa & Serretti 2009; Khoury et al. 2015). This has the added benefit of providing a substance-free aid to inspiration: open-monitoring forms of meditation induce divergent-thinking states that promote creativity (Colzato et al. 2012). All of these methods will also help with regulating the high emotional intensity associated with extreme intelligence.

To optimise personal performance it is furthermore necessary to find ways of regulating other typical corollaries of very high IQ such as perfectionism and multipotentiality that can lead to burnout as well as to underachievement. Perfectionism can prevent getting started on something because of a fear of failing, or prevent bringing something to completion because of never thinking it is good enough. With multipotentiality, apart from it being difficult to know which of many talents to prioritise, a pitfall is that having the capacity to do many things well often sees those with high IQ taking on so many things that they are incessantly over-busy but without being able to pursue any one of them to a fulfilling level of mastery. I have had clients who suddenly wake up to this in mid-life with regrets at what suddenly feel like misspent years and an urgency to find a core direction.

At the other extreme from doing too much, is doing too little. Laziness can develop out of lacking challenges and motivation. Paralysing procrastination can be part of laziness, or part of perfectionism, or it can relate to general difficulties with executive function. Executive function refers to various aspects of managing oneself that are necessary for success, such as competence in focus and attention, planning and organisation, cognitive flexibility, emotional regulation, and impulse control. Many resources can be found on all of these issues. A few examples are: on perfectionism – Stoeber (2018); on burnout – Leiter & Maslach (2005); on executive function – Honos-Webb (2018).

What is success?

In Chapter 6 we reflected on how benefit versus liability were defined. Now, in considering what constitutes thriving, it is pertinent to reflect on what we mean by "success". There is a tendency in the West to laud individualistic achievement as the most highly prized attainment, together with a tendency for portraying great achievements as being individualistic. People like to credit inventions and developments to one named "genius scientist" – like Isaac Newton – without fully recognising his or her assistants, collaborators, and influencers. Yet a study of 2,026 scientists (that included Newton) showed that the more eminent a scientist was, the more interactive links he or she had with other eminent scientists (Simonton 2009). Without Charles Darwin having friends who orchestrated the publication of his *On the Origin of Species* to precede that of a prior essay written by Alfred Wallace, it would have been Wallace who would have been given credit for originating the thesis of natural selection (Simonton 2009). Very often new ideas arise close together in time in different places, with those involved having to race to go down in history as that idea's creator.

The tendency towards lauding the individual exacerbates social problems around well-achieving high-IQ individuals by making others resent their heralded success precisely because others are not adequately recognised in their perhaps more modest, as well as collective, yet widely essential contributions and occupations. This constitutes an ignoring and devaluing of such supporting roles in favour of endorsing individual glory. Some supporting roles might conceal neglected forms of genius. For example, the intuitive, canny, and dedicated PAs of many big names, or the unsung nannies who helped raise high achievers or their children. There are no Nobel prizes for parenting. There is often an aim to find childcare – as though it is a mere chore – so as to enable a return to work as soon as possible, as though a professional career is where the real importance lies. Yet – as neuropsychological evidence emphasises – those early caregiving experiences, with their lifelong influence, are crucial for the wellbeing and successful functioning of every human being.

The individualistic-achievement mentality can translate into high-potential individuals only thinking they are being successful if they really do totally stand out from others and remain set apart, or they might feel a pressure to present themselves in this way. Grobman (2009) has written about how the process of therapy with highly gifted individuals included them having to come to see that functioning with complete autonomy was a myth to begin with, when recognising everyone else who had been involved in their lives and development. They also had to realise that the involvement of these others and acknowledgement of their involvement did not detract from their own individuality. Self-absorption had blinded them to their obvious dependency on others. They needed to drop their facade of independence and invincibility (Grobman 2009), which is a facade so easily adopted in the West where interdependence within a non-individualist community is a more foreign concept.

How success is defined can also change over time. Even collective achievements that are hailed as great successes of apparently extreme intelligence may later prove to have unforeseen detrimental – even catastrophic – consequences. An example is that modern mass agricultural practices, seen as the solution to guaranteeing constant national food supplies, have with their increasing technologisation, chemicalisation, and commercialisation wrought such destruction to natural ecosystems and indigenous community lifestyles that they have become a serious threat to the well-being and even the future of our planet and its inhabitants (see the Gaia Foundation's profound *We Feed the World* international project, searchable online). It took extreme intelligence, too, to invent an atom bomb, but does that count as a success?

Summary

This chapter has presented a few guiding principles on how high ability can be helped to thrive. When extreme intelligence is identified and information about its associated risks and vulnerabilities is understood, resources can be sought and strategies implemented that facilitate healthy psychosocial development and an actualising of potential. The importance of a balanced reaction to high potential, boundaries, affect regulation, psychoeducation, mentalisation, and effective communication has been highlighted for safeguarding against the naivety and arrogance that have been shown to underlie much interpersonal difficulty. The latter is, in turn, what underlies much wastage of potential. The change process involved in moving towards "Thriving" has been analysed, emphasising the benefits of improving interpersonal understanding and skill and experiencing relational repair of difficulty and despair. It has been highlighted that managing the dynamics of collaboration and competition effectively – as well as managing stress, perfectionism, and multipotentiality – is vital for supporting personal performance and combating the underachievement that plagues many very high-IQ individuals. The significance has also been pointed out of recognising collective contributions to success, as well as of questioning what constitutes success.

References

Booth, P. B. (2010). *Theraplay*. (3rd ed.). San Francisco, CA: John Wiley & Sons.

Chiesa, A. & Serretti, A. (2009). Mindfulness-based stress reduction for stress management in healthy people: a review and meta-analysis. *Journal of Alternative Complementary Medicine*, 15(5), pp. 593–600.

Colzato, L. S., Ozturk, A. & Hommel, B. (2012). Meditate to create: the impact of focused-attention and open-monitoring training on convergent and divergent thinking. *Frontiers in Psychology*, 3. Published online. doi: 10.3389/fpsyg.2012.00116.

Corten, F., Nauta, N. & Ronner, S. (2006). *Highly intelligent and gifted employees – Key to innovation?* (English translation). Academic paper delivered in Amsterdam, 11 October 2006 at International HRD-conference. [online] Available at: www.triplenine.org/articles/Nauta-200610.pdf. [Accessed 12 June 2012].

De Raat, F. (2002). Hoogbegaafdheid werkt niet altijd goed (Giftedness doesn't always work well). *NRC Handelsblad*. [online] Available at: www.xi2.nl/bronnen/hbwerkt.htm. [Accessed 12 June 2012].

Dweck, C. S. (2006). *Mindset: How You Can Fulfil Your Potential*. London: Constable & Robinson Ltd.

Fadda, R., Rapinett, G., Grathwohl, D., Parisi, M., Fanari, R., Calo, C. M. & Schmitt, J. (2012). Effects of drinking supplementary water at school on cognitive performance in children. *Appetite*, 59, pp. 730–737.

Farmelo, G. (2009). *The Strangest Man*. London: Faber & Faber.

Fonagy, P., Gergely, G., Jurist, E. L. & Target, M. (2004). *Affect Regulation, Mentalization, and the Development of the Self*. London: Karnac Books.

Fonseca, C. (2016). *Emotional Intensity in Gifted Students – Helping Kids Cope with Explosive Feelings*. (2nd ed.). Waco, TX: Prufrock Press.

Freeman, C. & Power, M. (2007). *Handbook of Evidence-Based Psychotherapies*. Chichester: Wiley.

Goleman, D. (1998). *Working With Emotional Intelligence*. London: Bloomsbury.

Gordon, W. (n.d.). *Help ... My Client is Brilliant! Coaching People with High IQs*. [online] Available at: http://downloads.mhs.com/ei/Coaching-High-IQ-Clients.pdf. [Accessed 7 February 2017].

Grobman, J. (2009). A psychodynamic psychotherapy approach to the emotional problems of exceptionally and profoundly gifted adolescents and adults: a psychiatrist's experience. *Journal for the Education of the Gifted*, 33(1), pp. 106–125.

Hiles Howard, A. R., Lindaman, S., Copeland, R. & Cross, D. R. (2018). Theraplay impact on parents and children with autism spectrum disorder: improvements in affect, joint attention, and social cooperation. *International Journal of Play Therapy*, 27(1), pp. 56–68.

Hodges, A. (2014). *Alan Turing: The Enigma*. London: Vintage Books.

Hollway, W. (2015). *Knowing Mothers: Researching Maternal Identity Change. Studies in the Psychosocial*. London: Palgrave Macmillan.

Honos-Webb, L. (2018). *Brain Hacks*. Emeryville, CA: Althea Press.

Hunt, E. (2011). *Human Intelligence*. New York: Cambridge University Press.

Isaacson, W. (2011). *Steve Jobs: The Exclusive Biography*. New York: Simon & Schuster.

Jacobsen, M.-E. (1999). *The Gifted Adult*. New York: Ballantine Books.

Khoury, B., Sharma, M., Rush, S. E. & Fournier, C. (2015). Mindfulness-based stress reduction for healthy individuals: a meta-analysis. *Journal of Psychosomatic Research*, 78(6), pp. 519–528.

Kusy, M. & Holloway, E. (2009). *Toxic Workplace: Managing Toxic Personalities and Their Systems of Power*. San Francisco, CA: Jossey-Bass.

Leiter, M. P. & Maslach, C. (2005). *Banishing Burnout*. San Francisco, CA: Jossey-Bass.

Lindsay, W. R. & Sturney, P. (2007). Intellectual disabilities. In: C. Freeman & M. Power (Eds.). *Handbook of Evidence-Based Psychotherapies*. Chichester: Wiley. pp. 193–214.

Menel, J. (2008). Multipotentiality in the workplace. *Mensa Research Journal*, 39(2), pp. 40–46.

Mollon, P. (2001). *Releasing the Self – The Healing Legacy of Heinz Kohut*. London: Whurr Publishers.

Nauta, N. & Corten, F. (2002). Gifted adults in work (English translation). *Tijdschrift voor Bedrijfs- en Verzekeringsgeneeeskunde* (Journal for Occupational and Insurance Physicians), 10(11), pp. 332–335. [online] Available at: www.sengifted.org/archives/articles/gifted-adults-in-work. [Accessed 12 June 2012].

Nauta, N. & Ronner, S. (2013). *Gifted Workers Hitting the Target*. MaastrichtMaa: Shaker Media.

Perrone, K., Civiletto, C. & Webb, L. (2004). Perceived barriers to and supports of the attainment of career and family goals among academically talented individuals. *International Journal of Stress Management*, 11(2), pp. 114–131.

Persson, R. S. (2009). The unwanted gifted and talented: a sociobiological perspective of the societal functions of giftedness. In: L. V. Shavinina (Ed.). *International Handbook on Giftedness*. Quebec: Springer. pp. 913–924.

Peters, S. (2018). *My Hidden Chimp*. London: Studio Press Books.

Peterson, J. S. (2015). School counsellors and gifted kids: respecting both cognitive and affective. *Journal of Counseling & Development*, 93(2), pp. 153–162.

Peterson, J. S. & Moon, S. M. (2008). Counseling the gifted. In: S. I. Pfeiffer (Ed.). *Handbook of Giftedness in Children: Psychoeducational Theory, Research, and Best Practices*. New York: Springer. pp. 223–245.

Schore, A. N. (2012). *The Science of the Art of Psychotherapy*. New York: W. W. Norton & Company.

Silverman, L. K. (2013). *Giftedness 101*. New York: Springer.

Simonton, D. K. (2009). *Genius 101*. New York: Springer.

Stoeber, J. (Ed.). (2018). *The Psychology of Perfectionism*. New York: Routledge.

Streznewski, M. K. (1999). *Gifted Grown Ups: The Mixed Blessings of Extraordinary Potential*. New York: John Wiley & Sons.

Tan, C.-M. (2012). *Search Inside Yourself*. London: Harper Collins.

Towers, G. M. (1987). The outsiders. *Gift of Fire*, 22. [online] Available at: www.cpsimoes.net/artigos/outsiders.html. [Accessed 5 February 2017].

Webb, J. T., Amend, E. R., Beljan, P., Webb, N. E., Kuzujanakis, M., Olenchak, F. R. & Goerss, J. (2016). *Misdiagnosis and Dual Diagnoses of Gifted Children and Adults*. (2nd ed.). Tucson, AZ: Great Potential Press.

Weeks, H. (2008). *Failure to Communicate*. Boston, MA: Harvard Business Press.

Williams, S. (2017). How 12-year old Alma Deutscher became the world's "little Mozart". *The Telegraph*. [online] Available at: www.telegraph.co.uk/women/life/meet-prodigy-alma-deutscher-12-year-old-opera/ [Accessed 9 May 2019].

Yazdani, S. & Daryei, G. (2016). Parenting styles and psychosocial adjustment of gifted and normal adolescents. *Pacific Science Review B: Humanities and Social Sciences*, 2(3), pp. 100–105.

Yermish, A. (2010). *Cheetahs on the Couch: Issues Affecting the Therapeutic Working Alliance with Clients Who Are Cognitively Gifted*. Unpublished PhD thesis, Massachusetts School of Professional Psychology.

CONCLUSION

Implications for the world around us

> **Reflective Prompt 10:** Can you name one change that you would most like to see happen in the way that intelligence is currently dealt with in the world around you? This could relate to anything from the attitudes or behaviours of family, friends or colleagues to the procedures in schools or workplaces, depictions in the media, or government policy. Can you describe how you think this particular change would make a positive difference?

Having started the book by focusing on how we think and speak about extreme intelligence, we now return to this question. It stands to reason that if individuals at the far left edge of the Bell Curve need special attention because of how that affects their lives, this would be true too of people who are at least two standard deviations away from the norm at the far right extreme of human intelligence. However, such individuals are not usually thought of as living with an individual difference that has associated special needs. If such individuals show ineptness in practical or social matters, they are often mocked and vilified for it with some degree of glee – "so smart and yet so dumb!" – rather than shown respect and compassion for what the nature of their struggle is. And as there has now been research correlating very high IQ with a higher incidence of autism, this gives further evidence that an individual difference is present that needs attention not criticism. A person with low IQ and autism would be given assistance, not criticised for it.

It is interesting that we even speak differently of our observations at the Bell Curve's two extremes. We usually say someone *has* a learning disability, versus someone *is* gifted: the former suggests a whole person who happens to be contending with an intellectual deficit, whereas the latter suggests that the whole of the person is identified with their intellectual surplus. Language has evolved for the lower end of the intellectual spectrum, so that Binet's original terms such as "moron" and "imbecile" (Nicolas et al. 2013) are now considered inappropriate and have been replaced with the more scientifically descriptive term "learning disability". I think it is time for the upper end of the spectrum to evolve also, and for the term "gifted" to be seen as similarly inappropriate and outdated. I would put forward as an alternative my suggested term "learning agility".

A minority group means those who have less power, rather than necessarily being fewer in number, relative to other groups. Where those with extreme intelligence are concerned, they are definitely far fewer in number, and they also have less power than other groups when they are ignored, not suitably catered for – educationally, for example – and when discriminated against, stigmatised, and marginalised. However – and this is precisely wherein all the complication lies – they can also hold more power than the majority if they have successfully channelled their abilities and thereby gained positions of influence and privilege.

It is because high IQ is so much associated with elitism that it is hard for people to have compassion for the difficulties that those with extremely high IQ might experience. However, this – adapting Tolan's (1996) metaphor – is like saying of a cheetah with a wounded leg that we are not bothered about it because even with its wounded leg it might be able to manage to run as fast as other animals can. It is like saying that the cheetah being in pain and unable to make full use of its natural ability is not important because the priority is to try to help other animals to run faster. Or saying let the cheetah stay wounded and suffering because it is unfair that, if it was supported to be at its best, it would be able to outrun the other animals. High ability, influence, and privilege attract *Schadenfreude*, explicit envious attacks, and even pogroms that have massacred successful peoples worldwide including in the Soviet Union, Turkey, Africa, China, Cambodia, and Malaysia: as Pinker (2002:152) has documented, "many atrocities of the 20th century were committed in the name of egalitarianism". It is difficult for people to want to support policies or actions that are likely to lead to successes that – this is what the fear is – could in some way threaten their own prospects of flourishing and/or create even more social inequality. However, not investing support for extremely intelligent individuals to be at their best begets a loss to society of brilliant minds as well as a burden in high-IQ crime, substance abuse, and mental and physical ill health.

The reality is that – in spite of movements that have sought to deny that individual differences in intelligence even exist – individual differences in intelligence are neurobiological and largely genetically determined and are not going to go away through sufficient personal effort or correct social policy. What is key is not to be ignorant or repudiating of this reality, or to fall prey to discrimination in relation to it. What is needed is to work to genuinely understand and be responsive to the issues involved so as to promote equal compassion for every human being no matter where on the Bell Curve he or she might be placed, for the mutual benefit of all. Being able to recognise exactly how this is of mutual benefit for all is pivotal.

Members of government of countries as widespread as Germany and Indonesia have addressed international conferences on giftedness with urgings that, given the complexity of challenges facing us in the 21st century and the "finite natural and capital resources" of the world, the optimal preservation and development of "superior quality human resources" is needed, and that it is essential "that people with outstanding abilities and the willingness for excellence co-operate" (cited in Persson 2009). The SMPY project is an exemplar of the far-reaching positive outcomes that are possible when extremely intelligent individuals are nurtured to achieve their best: not only did one IQ-type selection test in early adolescence accurately identify potential, but also decades later the contributions the participants have produced include patents, publications, and the taking up of senior teaching and research posts far in excess of national averages (Clynes 2016). The designers of this project set out to nurture extremely intelligent youngsters precisely so as to "change the world" (Clynes 2016:153). Within the opportunity this project provided of suitable channels for ability, the participants displayed high levels of motivation including willingness to work more hours than others (Hunt 2011). While governments shy away from engaging with such potentials, the private educational sector continues to unabashedly select for and tailor provision specifically to highly able children, privileging those who can afford the steep tuition fees and thereby perpetuating a riven society. Now, more than ever, intelligence should be more widely valued and invested in – not for the glory of the individual, but for the collective good – because it is becoming a diminishing resource: the dysgenic trend and Negative Flynn Effect show that intelligence in developed countries is in decline.

Paraphrasing Leon Megginson's words on his reading of Darwin (Darwin Correspondence Project, n.d.), it is not the most intelligent of the species nor the strongest that survives, but the one that is able best to adapt to the changing environment in which it finds itself. Might autism – a condition on the increase – itself be a kind of adaptation to a changing world that is seeing humans increasingly interacting more with digital devices than with fellow humans? If IT skills, rather than social skills, are becoming prioritised then a condition like autism in which social interaction is underdeveloped in favour of strengths in interacting with technology and data could be adaptive. How might developments of this kind change humanity as we currently know it?

Another development to consider, is the impressive progress being made in the field of artificial intelligence. Computer programmes have already outperformed human champions in a number of games from chess to cryptic trivia (Bostrom 2014). Do we mind whether or not optimal intelligence resides primarily in humans? Professor Nick Bostrom, who is Director of the UK's Future of Humanity Institute and Strategic Artificial Intelligence Research Centre, asserts that we cannot underestimate the serious risk to our humanity of an artificial "superintelligence" (Bostrom 2014). He heavily stresses how crucial it is to equip humans who are properly cognisant of and knowledgeable about the dangers of this to be competent to guide the path forward.

How can we have a healthier attitude about extreme intelligence in humans? Can we, instead of feeling guilty about, ashamed of, or enviously attacking of it, celebrate and take pride in it? Are we willing to support it to thrive? The usual work of advocates of minority groups is to change perceptions that members of those groups are worse than others because of their differences, for example specific disabilities they may have. The work of advocates of extreme intelligence might have to be that of changing perceptions that individuals who are so affected are better than others because of specific abilities they have. A healthier attitude involves neither neglecting or denigrating extreme intelligence nor idealising it, but validating it as an individual difference that – as with any individual difference – when properly attended to improves life for those affected and those around them.

How any environment responds to manifestations of extreme intelligence clearly has powerful impact. However, extremely intelligent individuals themselves have a significant part to play in how that ongoing process of recognition and interaction between person and environment unfolds. It will help very high-IQ individuals to become enlightened about the kinds of differences that exist between themselves and the majority of others within general environments. This would include becoming more aware of how they are perceived by and are treating others; how they might be unintentionally perpetuating interpersonal trouble; and what can be done about this. A lot of this hinges on this book's main themes of danger versus safety, and being set apart versus belonging. If a highly able person is perceived as an adversary for the securing of needed resources, then he or she is treated as a particularly formidable threat and is related to with covert or overt hostility. If a highly able person can be perceived as an ally, then his or her driven, quick and capable qualities become an asset to the securing of protection and resources, and hostility or obstructiveness is not provoked. When seeking to achieve belonging and collaboration, it might be a matter of developing the interpersonal skill to prime in the other an "ally" rather than "adversary" interpretation of relational status. This requires a minimising of both naivety and arrogance. Learning about and deliberately practising empathy, mentalisation, and effective communication are mainstays that will aid any individual to thrive in any environment in the world as we currently know it.

Summary

This conclusion draws together the book's main themes of danger versus safety, related to being set apart from others and/or rejected versus belonging. The two extremes on the Bell Curve of intelligence have been revisited, considering what language is used for these and how the special needs of each are typically responded to. How the world and humanity as we know it is changing has been raised, given an increase in autism, progress in artificial intelligence, and a decline in human intelligence as evidenced by the dysgenic trend and Negative Flynn Effect. It has been argued that we should not neglect, denigrate, or idealise extreme intelligence but seriously invest in this diminishing resource for the benefit of high-IQ individuals and the world around them. Lastly, it has been suggested that very high-IQ individuals can themselves contribute to improving their positions by increasing their emotional intelligence and, when affiliation and collaboration are desired, priming in others an "ally" rather than "adversary" interpretation of relational status.

This book has sought to inform of the issues surrounding extreme intelligence, to engage with the predicaments it presents, and to consider the implications for affected individuals and the world around us of how we relate to this in the attitudes we hold and the decisions we make. It has throughout invited readers to consider personal histories, attitudes and reactions to the issues involved, to probe their related knowledge and values, and to chart changes in these as development continues personally and in the world around us.

References

Bostrom, N. (2014). *Superintelligence*. Oxford: Oxford University Press.

Clynes, T. (2016). How to raise a genius. *Nature*, 537, pp. 152–155.

Darwin Correspondence Project. (n.d.). *The Evolution of a Misquotation*. University of Cambridge. [online] Available at: www.darwinproject.ac.uk/people/about-darwin/six-things-darwin-never-said/evolution-misquotation. [Accessed 15 May 2019].

Hunt, E. (2011). *Human Intelligence*. New York: Cambridge University Press.

Persson, R. S. (2009). The unwanted gifted and talented: a sociobiological perspective of the societal functions of giftedness. In: L. V. Shavinina (Ed.). *International Handbook on Giftedness*. Quebec: Springer. pp. 913–924.

Pinker, S. (2002). *The Blank Slate*. London: Penguin Books.

Nicolas, S., Andrieu, B., Croizet, J.-C., Sanitioso, R. B., & Burman, J. T. (2013). Sick? Or slow? On the origins of intelligence as a psychological object. *Intelligence*, 41(5), pp. 699–711.

Tolan, S. S. (1996). *Is It a Cheetah?* [online] Available at: www.stephanietolan.com/is_it_a_cheetah.htm. [Accessed 11 September 2016].

APPENDIX

Explaining the research process that underpins the book

This Appendix provides a glimpse of the research process underpinning this book. Those who would like more depth and detail may refer to Falck (2017).

Although the book also draws on my professional consulting experience with high-IQ adults, it principally took form from my doctorate on giftedness (Falck 2017). For this I used a qualitative research design, employing Kathy Charmaz's (2006; 2014) Constructivist Grounded Theory research methodology and Wendy Hollway's (2008; 2015; 2016) Psychosocial research epistemology. My research gained ethical approval from the Metanoia Institute (in conjunction with Middlesex University) and British Mensa, and was carried out in accordance with the British Psychological Society's Ethical Principles for Conducting Research with Human Participants (2006).

The aim of Constructivist Grounded Theory is to construct original theory that is fully grounded in research data and contributes to a given field a way of representing or making better sense of something that is puzzling or underexplored. Charmaz (2014:228) cites the definition of theory as that which "states relationships between abstract concepts and may aim for either explanation or understanding". What I wanted to make better sense of was why there is a stereotype of high IQ being paired with interpersonal difficulty. I also wanted to understand what might make the difference between high-IQ individuals who do versus those who do not experience – or who have ceased to experience – such difficulty. My research question therefore was: how does interpersonal difficulty in high-IQ individuals arise; how is it perpetuated; and how can it be overcome?

Summary of Constructivist Grounded Theory (CGT) procedures

In essence the carrying out of CGT involves collecting data, analysing it, processing your thoughts about the data (termed "memo writing"), gathering further data to test out your developing thoughts (termed "theoretical sampling"), and then out of all of that constructing theory that encapsulates your findings. The theoretical products of my research are the "High-IQ Context" model (presented in Chapter 3), the "High-IQ Relational Styles" framework (Chapter 8), and the "Change towards 'Thriving'" diagram (Chapter 9). The latter two "products" include incorporation of the "Naive Child" and "Arrogant Emperor" conceptualisations (presented in Chapter 5). I will now show how my going through the steps of the CGT methodology created these theoretical products.

Data collection

I collected data using two research instruments – semi-structured interviews, and textual analysis. These were ideal for CGT, for which you collect "rich data" that are "detailed, focused, full" (Charmaz 2006:14). I interviewed 20 high-IQ adults (ten male, ten female) between the ages of 26 and 58 (M=38.7), originating from 11 countries. Undertaking 20 interviews is consistent with the recommendations of Creswell (2013:86), and Green & Thorogood (2009:120) who maintain that "the experience of most qualitative researchers is that … little that is 'new' comes out of transcripts after you have interviewed 20 or so people". The first 16 interviewees were recruited through British Mensa. The final four were not Mensa members and were recruited in accordance with the principles of theoretical sampling (described below). My textual analysis was carried out on material in books and journals relevant to the interpersonal relating of gifted/high-IQ individuals.

Quality control

The interviews showed a high degree of accordance with Kvale & Brinkmann's (2009) quality criteria for interviews. This includes, for example, a great extent of "spontaneous, rich, specific and relevant" interviewee replies (Kvale & Brinkmann 2009:164), and the interviewer throughout querying internal contradictions and checking and obtaining the interviewee's verification of meanings and understandings. My academic advisor, two academic consultants, and four "critical friends" (see Kember et al. 1997) critiqued the research as meeting the validity criteria of coherence (Stiles 1993) and grounding in examples (Elliott et al. 1999).

Analysing the data

In CGT the data that has been collected is analysed into themes, termed "codes" (Charmaz 2006). You start with open codes which are more general, then sort these into focused codes which are more specific. Table A.1 below shows the focused codes I arrived at for each part of the research question. So as to provide an audit trail (Gray 2009:516), the numbers alongside each focused code correspond to identically numbered files I hold that contain relevant

TABLE A.1 Research data focused codes

Research question	Research data focused codes
Arising of interpersonal difficulty	A1. High IQ qualities A2. Place of high IQ in identity A3. Importance of utilising abilities A4. Implications for well-being B1. Workplace satisfaction B2. Differences in place/context C1. Others recognising high IQ C2. Realising you're different C3. Effort and speed
Perpetuating of interpersonal difficulty	D1. Belonging or not belonging D2. Interpersonal difficulty D3. Transference from past to present
Overcoming of interpersonal difficulty	E1. Hiding self E2. Change of environment E3. Improving interpersonal understanding and skill

excerpts from the (anonymised) transcripts of the source interviews. By this system the associated raw data can easily be referred back to.

Memo writing

In CGT a device used for processing your thinking as you immerse yourself in the data is termed "memo writing" (Charmaz 2006). In writing memos you as researcher "catch your thoughts, capture the comparisons and connections you make, and crystallize questions and directions for you to pursue" (Charmaz 2006:72). Such memo writing involves not only thinking about the interviewees' comments and the texts read and analysed, but also about the researcher's reflexivity. Reflexivity entails considering your own position, experiences and reactions during the research process (e.g. see Hollway 2016). Below is an example, which shows how my memo writing involved processing an amalgamation of reading, reflexivity, professional practice, and research data:

Memo
My thoughts on the *Office Politics* book (James 2013) and how it relates to my research project, are mingled with my reflexivity. I'm thinking about, in my own life, examples of my naivety … in politics … And I think of the parallels with my target population, as also exemplified in my client TH. The gifted person thing of lack of artifice, honesty, strong moral integrity – the "child" of [interviewee Ana's] emperor analogy – and how this makes such a person disastrous at politics. There is definitely an angle here. What is it that makes a gifted person so "straightforward", so unable to read the complexities, and so resistant to accepting the complexities, of the ordinary dissimulation of human social intercourse? This relates to [such individuals'] difficulty with conversation, in so far as conversation often involves avoiding or concealing, rather than engaging with, real issues. And there is something about how this relates to emotional intelligence, and the Asperger's thing. A certain kind of intense, sensitive, naive person, not made for this world. But can they learn, and do they want to learn, to better adapt? And can I help? … The thing of being authentic, or learning skill that doesn't annihilate authenticity. But how purist is a gifted person, can they see the difference between learning skill and forgoing authenticity?

In CGT, when a code includes the actual words a research participant has used it is called an *"in vivo"* code (Charmaz 2014:134). In my case I constructed two *in vivo* theoretical concepts, because I took the "child" and "emperor" figures from the story about the emperor's new clothes that interviewee Ana referred to and came to name my conceptualisation of the two main orders of interpersonal difficulty in high-IQ adults as Naive Child and Arrogant Emperor (as explained in Chapter 5).

Constructing theory

In CGT, after the initial data analysis stages of open coding and focused coding are completed, a move is made into higher levels of abstract thinking with the creation of theoretical categories. During these procedures I was constantly ruminating, and writing memos, about how the different elements of the data related to each other. Holton (2010) describes needing to trust in the "power of preconscious processing for conceptual emergence". Table A.2 below shows the theoretical categories I distilled out of the focused codes.

Out of this I created a theoretical structure that shows how the above-presented research data codes and theoretical categories dynamically relate to each other. I called this the High-IQ Context model. A streamlined version of this appears together with explication in Chapter 3, but Figure A.1 shows each part of the model together with its original constitutive data codes.

TABLE A.2 Research data focused codes and theoretical categories

Research question	Research data focused codes	Theoretical categories
Arising of interpersonal difficulty	A1. High IQ qualities A2. Place of high IQ in identity A3. Importance of utilising abilities A4. Implications for well-being	**A. Person** (nature of the person)
	B1. Workplace satisfaction B2. Differences in place/context	**B. Environment** (nature of the environment)
	C1. Others recognising high IQ C2. Realising you're different C3. Effort and speed	**C. Recognition** (recognition by person and environment of their respective natures)
Perpetuating of interpersonal difficulty	D1. Belonging or not belonging D2. Interpersonal difficulty D3. Transference from past to present	**D. Interaction** (interaction between person and environment)
Overcoming of interpersonal difficulty	E1. Hiding self E2. Change of environment E3. Improving interpersonal understanding and skill	**E. Change** (person making a change)

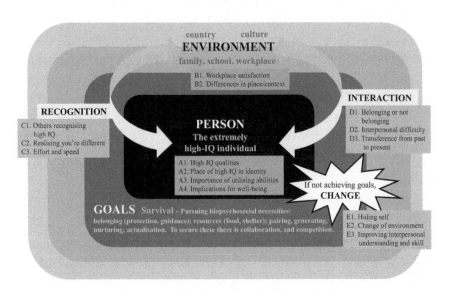

FIGURE A.1 High-IQ Context model with research data focused codes and theoretical categories

A Psychosocial interpretation of the data

What is presented in this Appendix so far comprises the readily accessible cognitive and behavioural aspects of my interviewees' interpersonal relating as reported to me by them. What I wanted to do next, was consider the more hidden, harder to articulate nuances of interpersonal experience, the unconscious processes that Psychodynamic and Systemic bodies of knowledge provide a language for but which is virtually unrepresented in the literature and research on high IQ/giftedness. Using a Psychosocial approach to interpret data is, as Hollway et al. assert (2005:179), "the best way of going beyond superficially descriptive" treatments of subjectivity. This would allow me to analyse the interesting links I had noticed between interviewees' developmental experiences and their current workplace experiences; how different individuals perceived and presented themselves differently in relation to their high IQ and interpersonal relations; and how all of this manifested in the way that the interviewee and I as interviewer interacted with each other.

I realised that to interpret these intersubjective aspects of the interviews I would need, as Hollway & Jefferson (2008) advocate, to look at each interview as a whole or gestalt. The traditional qualitative research technique of fragmenting the data from several interviews into codes and then reconstituting these fragments into an across-cases abstraction causes the data to lose its within-case coherence (Hollway & Jefferson 2008). I therefore went back and read through each original interview transcript again, making notes regarding the kinds of unconscious intersubjective processes I noticed. It is Chapter 7 that particularly engages with this content.

Theoretical sampling

After the above-described re-reading of each interview transcript as a whole, I wrote up a short interpretative story – like a brief case study – for each interview. Comparing these interpretative stories with each other allowed me to abstract from them the different styles of interpersonal relating that they evidenced. I condensed these general styles into a rough drafting of the four-quadrant High-IQ Relational Styles framework that is presented in completed form in Chapter 8. Further verifying these quadrants, before finalising them, was the next step.

In CGT, once your theorising is starting to take shape, you test it by undertaking "theoretical sampling" (Charmaz 2006). This is a method of gathering further data that specifically explores the directions your theorising is taking. To do this, I recruited and interviewed the final four research participants on the basis of each one appearing to have something in their lives relevant to one of the four quadrants. For example, over time, in a professional context, I noticed someone who seemed to keep moving away from securing the "top position" he was capable of, and who more than once mentioned his view that others might perceive him as "too big". I therefore invited him for interview to explore how he related to the "Inhibited" quadrant of the High-IQ Relational Styles framework I was theorising (which is presented in Chapter 8). With these final interviews I collected further data with which to probe the theory that was being constructed – to confirm the thinking, flesh it out, or challenge it. Throughout I was constantly comparing my existing data, the newly collected data, and my conceptual work (Holton 2010). I also used a talk I gave to Mensa members on 19 August 2016 as an opportunity to present my four-quadrant framework and test it out with an audience of high-IQ adults. It was enthusiastically received. How the textual analysis supports my theorising is presented particularly in Chapters 5 and 8. At this stage I could also finalise Figure 9.1 (Change towards "Thriving") which depicts the different kinds of change noticed in my interview data and how these relate to the Naive Child and Arrogant Emperor conceptualisations and the four quadrants of the High-IQ Relational Styles framework.

Limitations

The theory constructed in this project comprises a scholarly rather than a scientific contribution. Further research is being planned to test out the findings with a greater number of high-IQ adults.

I do not maintain that the theory presented in this project is exclusive to high-IQ individuals: many aspects are relevant to human beings in general at different times or to different degrees. However, with high-IQ individuals there is a predominance of certain kinds of experience because of their particular characteristics, and that is what my focus has been.

Wider applications

I have been asked whether my findings and models would be able to be applied to other minority groups. I cannot know this without undertaking similar research on other minority groups. I can see, however, that my High-IQ Context model (Chapter 3) could be used as a "blueprint" for dissecting the social development, predicaments, and implications of any other condition by examining how the existence of whatever that condition is becomes recognised by a person's environment, how this is noticed by the person themselves, and how the ensuing interactions between the person and their environment shape the person and can lead to changes being implemented, all within the overview of the biopsychosocial goals – starting with survival – that we as human beings seek to fulfil through our lifecourse. I can also see, in my High-IQ Relational Styles framework, that the dimensions in interpersonal relating that I have identified of expressiveness of self and acceptance by others, could be analysed in terms of how they play out in other minority groups. Anyone, and particularly a member of any minority group when faced with members of majority groups, will grapple with issues of how much it is safe to express of themselves and whether they will gain acceptance by others or not. However, how I have identified this as playing out in high-IQ individuals is uniquely grounded in my research data on this particular population.

Summary

This Appendix has summarised my qualitative research design involving semi-structured interviews and textual analysis. The methods of data collection and data analysis used have been described, as well as the processes unique to the Constructivist Grounded Theory methodology of memo writing, theoretical sampling, and the constructing of original theory. I have outlined my innovation of combining with this methodology a Psychosocial interpretation of the data, and included brief mention of research ethics, quality control, and the limitations of the project, as well as its potential wider applications.

References

British Psychological Society. (2006). *Ethical Principles for Conducting Research with Human Participants*. [pdf]

Charmaz, K. (2006). *Constructing Grounded Theory*. London: Sage.

Charmaz, K. (2014). *Constructing Grounded Theory*. (2nd ed.). London: Sage.

Creswell, J. W. (2013). *Qualitative Inquiry & Research Design – Choosing Among Five Approaches*. (3rd ed.). London: Sage.

Elliott, R., Fischer, C. T. & Rennie, D. L. (1999). Evolving guidelines for publication of qualitative research studies in psychology and related fields. *British Journal of Clinical Psychology*, 38, pp. 215–229.

Falck, S. (2017). *The Child, the Emperor, and the Fabulous Clothes: Constructing a Theory of How Interpersonal Difficulty in Gifted Adults Arises, is Perpetuated, and Can Be Overcome*. Unpublished dissertation submitted in partial fulfilment of the requirements for the Doctorate in Psychotherapy by Professional Studies at Metanoia Institute/Middlesex University.

Gray, D. E. (2009). *Doing Research in the Real World*. (2nd ed.). London: Sage.

Green, J. & Thorogood, N. (2009). *Qualitative Methods for Health Research*. (2nd ed.). Thousand Oaks, CA: Sage.

Hollway, W. (2008). The importance of relational thinking in the practice of psycho-social research: ontology, epistemology, methodology and ethics. In: S. Clarke; P. Hoggett & H. Hahn (Eds.). *Object Relations and Social Relations*. London: Karnac, pp. 137–162.

Hollway, W. (2015). *Knowing Mothers: Researching Maternal Identity Change. Studies in the Psychosocial*. London: Palgrave Macmillan.

Hollway, W. (2016). Emotional experience plus reflection: countertransference and reflexivity in research. *The Psychotherapist*, 62, pp. 1–6.

Hollway, W. & Jefferson, T. (2008). The free association narrative interview method. In: L. M. Given (Ed.). *The SAGE Encyclopedia of Qualitative Research Methods*. Sevenoaks, CA: Sage, pp. 296–315.

Hollway, W., Jefferson, T., Spears, R. & Wetherell, M. (2005). Panic and perjury: a psychosocial exploration of agency/commentary. *The British Journal of Social Psychology*, 44, pp. 147–163.

Holton, J. A. (2010). The coding process and its challenges. *Grounded Theory Review*, 9(1). [online] Available at: http://groundedtheoryreview.com/2010/04/02/the-coding-process-and-its-challenges/ [Accessed 15 January 2017].

James, O. (2013). *Office Politics*. London: Vermilion.

Kember, D., Ha, T.-S., Lam, B.-H., Lee, A., Ng, S., Yan, L. & Yum, J. C. K. (1997). The diverse role of the critical friend in supporting educational action research projects. *Educational Action Research*, 5(3), pp. 463–481.

Kvale, S. & Brinkmann, S. (2009). *Interviews – Learning the Craft of Qualitative Research Interviewing*. (2nd ed.). London: Sage.

Stiles, W. B. (1993). Quality control in qualitative research. *Clinical Psychology Review*, 13(6), pp. 593–618.

INDEX

Abagnale, Frank 89
ability 34
abstract thinking 22
acceptance by others 155–156, 158, 159, 161, 206–207
accreditations 76–77
ADHD *see* Attention-Deficit Hyperactivity Disorder
addiction 117; *see also* substance use
adjustment strategies 163
adolescents 54, 98, 110, 158, 168
affect regulation 133, 176–177; *see also* co-regulation; self-regulation
Agassi, Andre 133
age 34, 41
alcohol 40, 117, 119, 120
alienation 107, 116, 169; *see also* isolation; outsider; separation
alikeness 81
aloneness 107; *see also* isolation
amygdala 130
anger 35, 160
anti-intellectualism 17
anxiety 54, 83, 126, 151–152, 159, 174–175
apartheid 16, 42
Araoz, C. F. 118
Armed Services Vocational Aptitude Battery (ASVAB) 23
Armstrong, D. 60
arrogance 15, 103–104, 178; change in person-environment interaction 182, 184; minimisation of 198; narcissism 128, 129, 130–131; provoking 159
"Arrogant Emperor" profile 103–104, 105–107; arrogance in interpersonal relating 130–131; Narcissistic Personality Disorder 122, 127–129; provoking 159; research process 203; similarity with Naive Child 129–130
artificial intelligence 197–198
Asperger's syndrome 123–124
asynchrony 57, 100
atheism 59
atom bomb 192
attachment relationships 132–133, 134, 167–168
attachment styles 53, 100, 108, 167–169
Attachment Theory 52, 53–54, 55, 167
Attention-Deficit Hyperactivity Disorder (ADHD) 121, 122
augmentative approaches 38, 45
Australia 90
Auticon 179
autism/Autism Spectrum Disorder (ASD) 122–127, 130–131, 132, 134, 175, 177, 179, 195, 197, 199
avoidant attachment 100, 108, 167, 168

Bach, J. S. 25
Baddeley, Alan 23
Baker, H. S. 168
Baker, M. N. 168
Baron-Cohen, Simon 124

Index

Baumeister, R. F. 54
Beethoven, Ludwig van 25
Bell Curve 1–3, 5, 98, 116, 195
belonging 92, 127, 131–132, 198;
  Attachment Theory 53; evolutionary perspective 54; High-IQ Context model 52, 67; instinct of wanting to belong 166; separation versus 81–85
Benjamin, Jessica 55, 165, 177
Berlioz, Hector 115
Berne, Eric 151, 160, 167
Bettelheim, B. 125
Bick, E. 125
Binet, Alfred 18, 20, 21–22, 25, 28, 196
Bion, W. 149
Bipolar Disorder 119, 122
Blake, William 120
Blind Variation Selective Retention (BVSR) theory 119
boasting 14
Boccioa, C. M. 88, 89
bonding 132–133, 176–177
boredom 77, 88, 105, 121, 174
Bostrom, Nick 45, 197–198
boundaries 177–178
Bowlby, John 53
brain damage: disease 27, 40, 43, 44, 120; environmental toxins 40, 44; head injury 21, 40; brain function 39, 40, 54; "amygdala-highjacking" 130; autism 124–125; IQ tests 24; left and right hemispheres 120–121, 126; mother-infant interactions 126; primary and secondary process thinking 120–121
brain imaging 24, 37, 39, 126
brain integration 121; Parieto-Frontal Integration Theory (PFIT) 39
brain structure 39, 40, 45; cranial capacity 39; grey matter volume 24, 39; white matter density 39
breastfeeding 44
Brinkmann, S. 201
bullying 61, 76, 84, 85, 142–143; interpersonal difficulties 97, 108, 109; long-term effects 159
burnout 190

Carroll, John 19
Casement, P. 152
Catch Me If You Can (film) 89
Cattell-Horn theory 19, 24
Cattell-Horn-Carroll (CHC) theory 19
Cattell, Raymond Bernard 18, 19, 24
ceremonies 76

change 51–52, 65–66, 151–152, 153, 181–187; *see also* resistance to change
Charlton, B. G. 101
Charmaz, Kathy 106, 200
Chaudoir, S. R. 110
cheetah metaphor 26–27, 196
chess 36
children: asynchronous development 57; attachment relationships 132–133, 167–168; comparing and competing 74–75; identification of extreme intelligence 174–175; interpersonal difficulties 97, 98, 99–100; narcissism 128; parental pressure 35; praising 87; resources 175–176; secure base 133–134; strategies 176–178; *see also* infants
Chinese culture 62, 77
chronometrics 24, 37
Churchill, Winston 16
Cicoria, Tony 42–43, 120
co-regulation 53–54, 133, 134, 176–177; *see also* affect regulation; self-regulation
coaching 188
Cognitive-Behavioural Therapy 55, 167
Cohn 109
Coleman, L. J. 109, 166
collaboration 55, 192; High-IQ Context model 52, 67; presenting as an ally 198, 199; thriving 161; workplaces 178, 179–180, 181
Columbus Group 57
common sense 101
communication difficulties 107, 122
comparison 74–75
compassion 90–91, 189, 195, 196–197
competition 55, 74, 92, 192; High-IQ Context model 52, 67; lack of 87; natural competitiveness 75; sibling rivalry 148; thriving 161; workplaces 180
complacency 64
complexity 100
computer analogy 45–46
confidence 64, 87, 103, 127–128, 129
conflicts 107
constraints 26–27
Constructivist Grounded Theory (CGT) 200–204, 205–206
containment 177
contempt 129, 131–132
Corten, F. 160, 163, 164, 165
Coyle, D. 4
creativity 8, 57, 118–121, 179, 190
Crespi, B. J. 124, 125

Creswell, J. W. 201
criminal behaviour 88–89, 105, 116, 158, 196
CRISPR/Cas9 43
Cross, T. L. 110, 158
crystallised intelligence (Gc) 19, 24, 42, 45, 96
cultural bias 24
cyborgs 38–39, 45

Dabrowski, Kazimierz 57, 125
danger 66–67, 73, 198
Darwin, Charles 16, 18, 119, 191, 197
defences 54–55
degradations 76–77
denial 80
depression 59, 119, 158, 159, 166, 174–175
"deservingness" 90
despair 155, 158–159, 162–163, 164, 181, 184–185
Detterman, D. K. 99
Deutscher, Alma 176
"deviance fatigue" 109
Diagnostic and Statistical Manual of Mental Disorders (DSM) 33, 123, 126, 129, 132
diagnostic categories 121–122
Dirak, Paul 190
disabled children 168
discrimination 17, 21, 26, 41, 42, 110, 196
disdain 88, 89
disease 120
disinhibition 120
"divergency" 106
divergent thinking 120, 176, 190
Diversity Wheel 34
DNA 39–40; *see also* genetics
dreams 119–120
Drews, Elizabeth 164
drive 100
drug use 116, 117, 119, 120, 196
DSM *see Diagnostic and Statistical Manual of Mental Disorders*
dual exceptionality 5, 23, 26, 100, 132, 174, 175; *see also* multiple exceptionality
"dumbing down" 62, 65, 145
Dweck, C. S. 18, 87
dysgraphia 174
dyslexia 23, 175

Eastern bloc countries 61–62
education 41, 118; educational brands 46; eleven-plus 32; IQ linked to qualifications 25–26; private sector 197; selection policies 32; *see also* schools

effort 79–80, 85–87, 90
egalitarianism 196
Einstein, Albert 25, 121
Elgar, Edward 133
elitism 15, 196
emotional intelligence 100, 118, 178, 199
emotional intensity 57, 174, 190
empathy 124, 198
engaging with the world 58
environment 40, 60; bias towards environmental explanations of intelligence 47; changing the environment 63–64, 65–66, 181–182, 183–184; computer analogy 46; environmental toxins/pollutants 40, 44; High-IQ Context model 51–52, 206; improving intelligence 44–45; nature versus nurture debate 36, 38; person-environment interaction 60–63, 65, 66, 182, 184–187; twin studies 40–41
envy 91, 101, 144, 196
Erickson, Lisa 110
Ericsson, Anders 33, 34, 35, 36
Erikson, Erik 53, 75, 163
Esping, A. 13, 17
ethics 37, 38, 43, 44, 45, 47, 200, 207
ethnicity 34, 42, 46, 60; *see also* race
eugenics 16, 21, 32, 43, 44
evolutionary perspective 54, 59
evolutionary psychology 59
executive function 190
exercise 190
expectations 60, 63–64, 65, 106, 129, 153
expertise 4, 5, 7, 33, 35, 85
expressiveness of self 155–156, 158, 159, 161, 181–182, 206
extreme intelligence: attitudes to 195–198; autism 123–125, 126; being set apart versus belonging 81–85; biological basis 56, 58; criminal behaviour 88–89; definition of 2–3, 56; development of 8; effort and achievement 85–87; environment 60–65; experiential and behavioural characteristics 57, 58; False Self 166; goals 59–60; hiding 91–92, 110, 155, 156–159; High-IQ Context model 51–52, 67, 203–204, 206; High-IQ Relational Styles framework 154–169, 181–182, 205–206; hostility towards 90–91, 101, 107–108, 160, 173, 198; identification of 174–175, 187, 192; IQ scores 26, 56; minority status 57–58; Narcissistic Personality Disorder 127–129; nature versus nurture debate

32–37; psychosocial aspects 7; recognition 75–78; social difficulties 8, 95–111, 130; threats 173; *see also* giftedness; IQ
eye contact 124
Eysenck, Hans 18, 120

"fade-out effect" 44
False Self 166, 167, 181
family environments 61, 86; *see also* parents
Favier-Townsend, A. 6, 86–87, 159
Feather, Norman 90
Fiedler, E. 158, 163
Fisher, J. D. 110
fluid intelligence (*Gf*) 19, 24, 42, 45, 96
Flynn Effect 43, 47; *see also* Negative Flynn Effect
Fonagy, P. 129, 185
Fonseca, C. 178
Freeman, Joan 83, 95, 97, 157, 160
Freud, Sigmund 74, 128, 142, 145, 149, 167

g (general factor of intelligence) 19, 23, 116, 169
Gagné, F. 4, 33, 35, 85
Gaia Foundation 192
Gale, C. R. 119
Galton, Francis 5, 16, 18, 25, 32, 38, 119
Gardner, Howard 18, 19–20, 27, 38
Garfinkel, H. 76
Gates, Bill 36
"geek", definition of 130–131
gender 22, 23–24, 26, 34, 60, 62
general intelligence (*g*) 19, 23, 116, 169
genes 40, 43–44
genetic engineering 43–44
genetics 32, 38, 39–40, 41, 47, 124, 196
genius 7, 24–25, 36, 118–121, 132, 134
Genome-wide Complex Trait Analysis (GCTA) 39
Ghiselli, E. E. 118
giftedness: awareness of 165; biological basis 56; children 74; definition of 4; divergent thinking 176; effort and speed 85; experiential and behavioural characteristics 57; hiding 110; identification of 26; interpersonal difficulties 97–99; IQ scores 2; minority status 57–58; Narcissistic Personality Disorder 127–129; neural efficiency 39; research 7; as a special educational need 87; stereotypes about 95, 110; therapeutic treatment 188–189;

unwanted 109; use of the term 5, 14, 195–196; *see also* extreme intelligence
"giftophobia" 110
Gimbernat, A. 148–149
Girard, L.-C. 44
Gladwell, Malcolm 4, 33, 36
goals 52–55, 59–60, 206
"God syndrome" 89, 103
Goleman, D. 130
Gould, Stephen Jay 32–33, 34–35
Grandin, T. 125
grandiosity 128, 129, 177
Green, J. 201
Grobman, Jerald 87, 95, 129, 157, 175, 177, 187, 191
groups 41–42, 148–149
growth-oriented mindset 177
Guenole, F. 97, 98
guilt 35, 80–81, 109, 157, 186, 187

habits 63–64, 65, 87, 152, 153
Haier, R. J. 6, 13, 24, 44, 120
Hambrick, D. Z. 35
Hamilton, Alexander 89
Hardy, G. H. 119, 133
Harry Potter 96
Hawking, Stephen 27
Hayes, Tom 89, 103
Head Start 44
Hearst, Caroline 124, 125, 126, 127
helping others 180
heritability 39–40, 41; *see also* genetics
Hermione Granger 96
Herrnstein, Richard 26, 32–33
Hiding Self 155, 156–159, 162, 166, 167, 169, 181
Hierarchy of Needs 53
High-IQ Context model 51–52, 67, 203–204, 206
High-IQ Relational Styles framework 154–169, 181–182, 205–206
historiometrics 25
Hitler, Adolf 42
Hollingworth, Leta 5, 18, 98–99
Hollway, Wendy 54–55, 200, 205
Holton, J. A. 203
homophily 81, 127, 131–132
homosexuality 126, 132
Honos-Webb, L. 190
Horn, John 19, 24
Horta, B. L. 44
Horton, R. S. 128
hostility 90–91, 101, 107–108, 160, 173, 198

Howe, D. 168
Howe, M. J. A. 33
hubris 14, 31, 89, 132
human-machine integration 38–39
human worth 15, 16, 17
Humanistic approach 53, 55
humour 185
Hunt, E. 21, 26, 27, 85

Ibbotson, E. 96
ICD *see International Statistical Classification of Diseases*
identity 110, 150, 151
imagination 122
impatience 103, 104, 105
"imposter syndrome" 87
in vitro fertilisation (IFV) 43
incomes 25–26, 41
indignance 159–160, 169, 186–187
individual differences 16, 33–34, 196, 198; environmental factors 47; nature versus nurture debate 36; neurodiversity 126; understanding 185
individualism 190–191
infants 53–54, 55–56, 61, 125–126, 133; *see also* children
Ingram, P. 81
inhibition 155, 156–157, 163, 164, 181
innateness 32–33
insecure attachment 100, 167, 168–169
intellectual disability 2, 34
"intellectual neglect" 86–87, 159
intelligence: and ageing 42; appraisal of 26–28; Bell Curve 1–3, 195; computer analogy 45–46; controversial nature of 5, 13, 14–17, 28; definitions of 14, 17–18, 37, 38–39; group differences in 22, 38, 42; identification of 25–26; increasing 37–38, 43–44; language of 3–5; measurement of 20–25, 37; and musical taste 59; and political affiliation 59; and religious preference 59; research 5–7, 37–45; theories of 18–21; *see also* extreme intelligence; IQ
intelligence testing 20–25; *see also* IQ tests
intensity 57, 100, 174, 190
interaction 7, 8, 39, 43, 51–55, 60, 63, 65, 96, 98, 107, 109, 110, 122, 124, 126, 130, 142, 147–149, 151, 154, 159, 165, 166, 168, 169, 175, 177, 197, 198, 204, 206; *see also* interpersonal interaction
internal working models 53, 151, 167
International Society for Intelligence Research (ISIR) 116

International Statistical Classification of Diseases (ICD) 123
interpersonal interaction 7, 8, 130–131, 132–133; change in person-environment interaction 182, 184–187; High-IQ Relational Styles framework 154–169; infants 55–56; interpersonal competence 118, 165; interpersonal difficulties 95–111; perpetuation of interpersonal trouble 141–153; research process 200, 202; threats 173; workplaces 178, 179; *see also* social difficulties
intersubjectivity 52, 54, 125–126
introversion 108
invisibility 109, 166
iodine deficiency 44
IQ: autism 124–125, 195; cognitive performance 57; criminal behaviour 88–89; definition of extreme intelligence 56; environmental influences 44–45; Flynn Effect 43; goals 59–60; High-IQ Context model 51–52, 67, 203–204, 206; High-IQ Relational Styles framework 154–169, 181–182, 205–206; interpersonal difficulties 95, 98–100, 200; iodine deficiency 44; minority status 57; Narcissistic Personality Disorder 127–128; need for supporting skills and traits 118; origin of concept 22; person-environment interaction 60–61; professional success 74, 116; research process 6–7, 200–207; self-recognition 78; *see also* intelligence
IQ tests 22–26, 28, 37, 76; Bell Curve 1–3, 5; chess 36; giftedness 5; identification of extreme intelligence 175; intellectual disability 34; relativity 27; discrepancy between verbal and performance/non-verbal scores 22, 98, 124, 175
Isaacs, E. B. 44
isolation 73, 99, 108, 132, 165; *see also* alienation; outsider; separation
IT skills 197
IVF *see* in vitro fertilisation

Jackson, Michael 133
Jacobsen, M.-E. 58, 100, 163, 164, 187
James, William 18, 118
Jamison, Kay Redfield 118, 119, 121
Jefferson, T. 54–55, 205
Jensen, Arthur 18, 99
job performance 21
Jobs, Steve 81–82, 97, 190

214 Index

John Hopkins University Centre for Talented Youth 117
Jones, T. W. 97

Kamin, Leon 18, 32, 34–35
Kanazawa, S. 13, 15, 16, 17, 26, 59, 101
Kanner, Leo 125–126
Karpinski, R. I. 118, 125
Kaufman, S. B. 33, 74
Kaufmann, F. A. 108
Kerr 109
knowledge 22, 32
Koestler, A. 120
Kohut, Heinz 81, 169
Kvale, S. 201

Lawrence, Caroline 31
laziness 64, 87, 190
leaders 116, 148
learning 109, 122, 176; ease and speed of 85; High-IQ Context model 51–52; "need for cognition" 59; passion for 57, 58
learning disability 2, 124, 195–196
Leary, M. R. 54
Leiter, M. P. 190
Lereya, S. T. 159
liberalism 59
life-stages model 75, 163
lightning, struck by 42, 120
Lindsay, W. R. 188
Loden, M. 34
Lovecky, D. V. 106
Lubin, D. B. 110
luck 36

Mackintosh, N. J. 26
Mae, Vanessa 35
Mandela, Nelson 109–110
manic-depressive illness *see* Bipolar Disorder
Maslach, C. 190
Maslow, Abraham 53
McQueen, Lee Alexander 134
meditation 190
Megginson, Leon 197
Meier, E. 59
Meltzer, D. 125
memo writing 202–203
memory 22, 33, 36, 44
Mendel, Gregor Johann 28
Mendick, R. 34
Menel, J. 179
Mensa 6, 56, 92, 100, 123, 150, 188, 201
mental age 21–22, 25

mental health problems 59, 116, 118–121, 132, 196; children 178; "intellectual neglect" 87; personal change 65; qualitative research 98; *see also* psychopathology
mentalisation 129–130, 185–186, 198
microaggressions 158–159
Millay, Edna St Vincent Millay 133
Miller, Alice 129, 167
mindset, fixed and growth 177
minority group 124, 196, 198, 206
minority status 57–58
Miranda, Lin-Manuel 89
mirroring 55, 125, 165–166, 169, 176–177
misbehaviour 75, 77, 88, 128
misdiagnosis 121–122, 132
misunderstandings 101, 104, 107, 132
Mollon, P. 169
Moodley, R. 110
Morris, M. W. 81
mother-infant interactions 126, 133, 168
motivation 27, 36, 57, 197
Mozart effect 6, 44
Mozart, Wolfgang Amadeus 25, 120, 121, 133
Mueller, C. M. 87
multiple exceptionality 5, 23, 26, 100, 132, 174, 175; *see also* dual exceptionality
multiple intelligences 19–20
multipotentiality 57, 101, 190
Murray, Charles 26, 32–33
music 36, 59, 120
Musk, Elon 96–97, 121, 176

"Naive Child" profile 103, 104–105, 106–107; Autism Spectrum Disorder 122–127; naivety in interpersonal relating 130–131; provoking 159; research process 203; similarity with Arrogant Emperor 129–130
naivety 102, 106, 130–131, 178; autism 123; change in person-environment interaction 182, 184; learning deficits 122; minimisation of 198; provoking 159
narcissism 127–129, 130–131, 132
Narcissistic Personality Disorder (NPD) 122, 127–129
National Autistic Society 125, 126
natural selection 16, 191
nature versus nurture 32–37, 38, 41
Nauta, N. 163, 164, 165
"need for cognition" 59
Negative Flynn Effect 43, 47, 197, 199
Neihart, M. 98

nemesis 14, 89, 132
"nerd", definition of 130–131
neural efficiency 39
neural imaging *see* brain imaging
neurodiversity 34, 126
Newton, Isaac 191
Nobel Prizes 32, 42, 191
nutrition 43, 44, 189

Object Relations 52, 55, 167
Obsessive Compulsive Disorder (OCD) 122
obstruction 108
offence, causing 102–103, 104
omega-3 44
Ossorio, P. G. 76
outsider 82, 92, 107, 142, 146, 169, 184; *see also* alienation; separation

Paganini, Niccolò 115
"pain of contrast" 152, 153
Panek, R. 125
parents: attachment relationships 132–133, 167–168; autistic children 125–126; being held back by 84–85, 90, 143–144, 146; early caregiving experiences 191; identification of extreme intelligence 174–175; narcissistic children 128–129; pressure from 35; resources 175–176; socioeconomic status 41; strategies 176–178; Tiger Mother 35, 46, 133; *see also* family environments
Parieto-Frontal Integration Theory (PFIT) 39, 121
past experiences 142–145, 146–148, 149–150, 152–153
perceiving the world 58
perfectionism 100, 190, 192
performance 3–4, 17, 32; computer analogy 45; intelligence testing 21; optimisation of 189–190; relative to others 57, 58
Perrone, K. 178
Person-Centred approach 167
person-environment interaction 60–63, 65, 66, 182, 184–187
personality characteristics 100, 117
Persson, Roland 108, 109–110, 149, 163, 164, 165
Peters, S. 178
Peyre, H. 98
PFIT *see* Parieto-Frontal Integration Theory
Picasso, Pablo 133
Pinker, S. 34, 196
Plath, Sylvia 118

Plato 15, 18
Plucker, Jonathan 13, 17–18
Pollock, Jackson 118
polymaths 57
potential 3–4, 134; actualisation of 108–109, 156, 157, 161, 162, 164, 168, 182; disavowal of 158, 164; wastage of 192
power 88, 90–91, 106, 196
practise 32, 33, 36, 42
praise 14, 75, 76, 87, 92, 177
prefrontal cortex 120–121, 130
primary process thinking 121
problem solving 141–142
professional success 25–26, 74, 116, 117, 118, 161
provoking 151, 155, 159–161, 162–163, 164, 167, 169, 182
Psychoanalytic approach 125, 167
Psychodynamic approach 55, 111, 128, 151–152, 205
psychopathology 8, 118–119, 132; Autism Spectrum Disorder 122–127; diagnostic categories 121–122; Narcissistic Personality Disorder 127–129; *see also* mental health problems
psychosis 120
Psychosocial approach 200, 205
psychosocial stages 163; *see also* Erik Erikson
psychosocial subjects 54–55
psychoticism 120

qualitative research 6–7, 98, 200–207

race 16, 23–24, 26, 34, 42; *see also* ethnicity
racism 15
rage 169
"rage to master" 59, 65
Ramanujan, Srinivas 119–120, 133
Ravenhill, Mark 152–153
Raven's Progressive Matrices 22, 24
Reaching Out 155, 159–161, 162, 182
reactions 76, 102, 198; past experiences 142; provoking 151, 159–161, 182
"reaction range" 40, 45
reading 58
reasoning 22
recognition 75–78, 151, 165–166, 198; High-IQ Context model 51–52, 67; infant-caregiver relationship 55–56; self-recognition 78–81
rejection 67, 97, 107, 110, 173; despair 158; fear of 54, 83, 132, 166; infants 52; intelligence testing 21; provoking 161

relational styles 154–169, 181–182, 205–206
Remington, Anna 124
Renzulli, Joseph 18, 57
repair 186, 192
repetition compulsion 149–151, 186
reproduction 16, 43, 54, 59; have children 6; childless 185
research 5–7, 17, 37–45, 200–207
resistance to change 151–152, 153
resources 36, 175–176, 186, 192
Ritchie, S. J. 15
Rogers, Carl 167
Roosevelt, Theodore 74
Rosener, J. 34
Rowling, J. K. 96

safety 53, 54, 66–67, 73, 84, 161, 198
SAT tests 23, 38, 85
Savanna Principle 59
savants 36, 121
Schadenfreude 75, 90, 91, 101, 196
schools: impact of past experiences 145; person–environment interaction 61, 62; recognition 77–78; resources 175–176; selective 85; transition to university 63; *see also* education
Schopenhauer, Arthur 97
Schore, A. N. 133
Schumann, Robert 118
Schwartz, W. 76
secondary process thinking 120–121
secure attachment 167, 168
secure base 53, 133–134, 161
selective schools 85
self-actualisation 53
self-concept 76–77, 87, 150
self-control 116
self-esteem 77, 87, 90–91, 127–128, 187; "Arrogant Emperor" profile 104; children 75; environmental influences 60; identity 151; "intellectual neglect" 159; low 35, 59, 108, 159, 169; mirroring 165–166; parent–child interaction 168; True Self 167; workplace roles 180
self-recognition 78–81
self-regulation 125, 133, 134; *see also* affect regulation; co-regulation
SENG (Supporting the Emotional Needs of the Gifted) conference 110
separation 53, 81–85, 151, 198; *see also* alienation; isolation; outsider

sexual orientation 16, 34; *see also* homosexuality
Shakespeare, William 25
Shenk, D. 35
sibling rivalry 148
Sidis, William James 184
Silberman, Steve 126
Silverman, L. K. 116, 169, 174
Simonton, D. K. 18, 36, 118, 119
sleep 167, 190; falling asleep and creativity 119–120
SMPY *see* Study of Mathematically Precocious Youth
social difficulties 8, 95–111, 122, 124, 126, 130–131, 167, 175, 184; *see also* interpersonal interaction
Social Learning Theory 128
social skills training 126
sociocultural context 20, 27–28, 38, 109
socioeconomic status (SES) 23–24, 41, 60, 82, 84, 163
spatial ability 22, 24
Spearman, Charles 18, 19, 23
Spears, Britney 133
speed 22, 24, 57, 79–80, 85, 101
stability of intelligence 42–43
standing out 73, 78, 81
Stanford-Binet Intelligence Test 2, 20
Stanley, Julian 85, 117
Star Trek (television series) 39, 134
status 74, 75, 76
Steele, C. M. 23, 110
stereotype threat 23–24, 26–27, 110
stereotypes 95, 96–97, 109, 110
Stern, William 18, 22
Sternberg, Robert 18, 20, 27, 38
stigmatisation 109, 110, 132, 158, 196
Stoeber, J. 190
stress 190, 192
Streznewski, M. K. 161, 164, 165, 187
Study of Mathematically Precocious Youth (SMPY) 85, 117, 176, 197
Sturney, P. 188
substance use 116, 117, 119, 120, 196
success 190–192; *see also* professional success
suicidality 59, 118, 134, 158
superstition 14
support 36, 133
survival 52–53, 54, 55, 56, 74, 75, 165, 206
Suzuki, Shinichi 33, 34
Syed, M. 4
Systemic approach 111, 149, 205

talent 4
"tall poppies" phenomenon 90
Tannenbaum, A. J. 110
Terman, Lewis 18, 20, 22, 24–25, 98, 118
theoretical sampling 205–206
Theory of Mind 123, 129
therapy 187–189, 191
"Tiger Mother" 35, 46, 133; stage parent 35, 129
Thorogood, N. 201
thriving 155, 161, 162–163, 164, 166–167, 168, 181–182, 186–187
Tolan, S. S. 26, 196
Towers, G. M. 88, 99–100, 108, 161, 163, 184
Transactional Analysis 55, 167
transference 143–144, 145–146, 186
trauma 128, 158, 162–163, 184–185, 186–187
triarchic theory of intelligence 20
True Self 56, 166, 167, 181–182
Turing, Alan 96, 97, 132, 190
Tustin, F. 125
twice exceptionality *see* dual exceptionality
twin studies 39–41
"twinship transference" 81, 127, 169

unconscious processes 111, 142, 143–144, 152–153, 186
underachievement 87, 110, 159, 190, 192
university, transition to 63, 82–83

valency 149, 186
Van Beest, I. 54

Van Gogh, Vincent 28
Vance, A. 97, 121
verbal ability 22, 23, 124
"vicious circle of contempt" 129
visual-spatial ability 22, 23, 125, 176
"voluntary marginalisation" 108

Wallace, Alfred 191
Walter, Marie-Thérèse 133
Warne, R. T. 17, 47
"We Feed the World" 192
Webb, J. T. 97, 99, 122, 123–124, 126, 127–129, 141, 168, 183
Wechsler, David 18, 23
Wechsler Adult Intelligence Scale (WAIS) 22, 23
Wechsler Intelligence Scale for Children (WISC) 2, 23, 98
West, K. K. 168
Williams, K. D. 54
Wing, Lorna 122, 123
Winner, E. 59
Winnicott, Donald 55–56, 165–166, 167
withdrawal 108, 169
Woods, Tiger 133
Woolf, Virginia 118
workplaces 80, 84, 86, 142–143, 146–147, 178–181

Yerkes, Robert 18, 23
Yermish, A. 76, 151, 158–159, 189

"zone of tolerance" 99–100
Zuckerberg, Mark 117

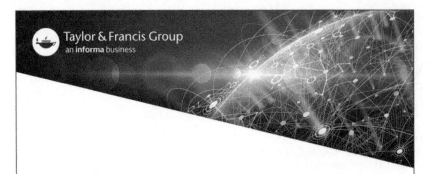